CONTENTS

CHAPTER 1: WHY YOU NEED THIS BOOK

It's The Only Soda Flavor Recipe Book Compatible with Popular Soda Makers

The home soda maker is a revolutionary invention because until now, soda was never thought to be a beverage that could be made at home. We enjoy soda at restaurants and in prepackaged cans and bottles, but there has never before been a simple, easy to use device that allows you to make sparkling water and many different sodas in the comfort of your own home. And the best part of the SodaStream is that it is so simple and easy to use that you will be making your own sodas minutes after you take it out of the box. This book will cover everything you need to know in order to become a soda making master, including in-depth instructions about how to make the perfect soda for your tastes, but also how to make create concoctions that will wow your guests. Our fun recipes will open up a whole new world of beverages that are sure to be surprising and refreshing.

Unlock Your Soda Maker's Potential for Amazing Sodas

Everyone has their own preference when it comes to the perfect soda. Some like sweet fruit flavors while others prefer traditional colas and root beers. Still others prefer the simple pleasure of a cold glass of sparkling water. Whatever your taste may be, the SodaStream is the perfect way to please everyone in your house. The problem with making your own soda has always been the same—how do you carbonate a beverage without lots of complicated equipment? This is why most people just buy soda and call it a day. But thanks to the SodaStream, there is no reason to compromise. The SodaStream offers a simple design that allows you to customize your beverage experience right down to the amount of carbonation in the drink. And since you are in control of the amount of carbonation and flavor, you will end up with the perfect tasting beverage every single time. The other great thing about the SodaStream is that since it has become the world's most popular at home soda making system, finding replacement CO_2 cartridges is inexpensive and easy.

Amazing Pro Tips for Making The Best Sodas You've Ever Had!

Let's face it, most of us don't have a lot of experience when it comes to making our own soda. Luckily, the SodaStream makes beverage making as easy as possible. In the pro tips section of this book, we will discuss the different ways that you can experiment with your SodaStream to create interesting and balanced flavors with just the right amount of carbonation. These industries approved tips will cover ways of blending natural flavors and sweeteners to make drinks that are creative and delicious. Why settle for store bought soda flavors when you can have exactly the flavor you want? Once you become an expert soda maker, you can impress your friends and family with fresh and exciting beverages that will become instant favorites. This section will cover everything you need to know in order to get the most out of your SodaStream so that you can keep experimenting every day.

Over 100 Delicious Recipes for Creative Sodas

Sure, there are some new flavors of soda out there, but most of us rely on a small rotation of classic sodas that have been around for generations.

Thanks to the SodaStream you can start thinking outside the box by creating sodas with flavors you've never thought of before. With over one hundred recipes for creative and refreshing sodas, this book will give you ideas to take your beverages to the next level.

It's The Only Soda Recipe Book You'll Ever Need

Not only does this book offer recipes and the science behind soda making, you will also learn how to consistently make a soda that fits your specific tastes. Big soda companies have been making soda the same way for decades, but now, thanks to the SodaStream you can make your own soda that rivals any can of soda on the market. And since the SodaStream is so easy to use and clean, you don't have any reason not to use it every day. We will also discuss how to make a simple refreshing glass of sparkling water that is a fun alternative to plain water and doesn't pack any extra calories. If you think about it, there's really no reason not to start making your own soda with the SodaStream today.

CHAPTER 2: HEALTH BENEFITS OF MAKING YOUR OWN SODA

Control Your Ingredients for Healthier Drinks

In recent years, we've heard a lot of new information about the health hazards of drinking too much soda. There are several reasons why so many people have become worried about their soda consumption, but luckily, the SodaStream allows you to continue to enjoy your favorite beverages, while cutting back on the ingredients that you may want to avoid. Since the SodaStream allows you to control the ingredients that go into your beverages, you don't have to consume anything you don't want to. And since plain sparkling water can be an excellent, refreshing alternative to still water, you don't even need to add any flavors to your water to have a fun and thirst quenching drink.

Sparkling Water Is a Great Alternative to Regular Soda

Sparkling water is a refreshing change of pace from traditional water, but it can also be a healthy way to drink fewer sugary beverages. But when faced with the high price of sparkling water at the grocery store, it hardly seems worth it. Thanks to your SodaStream you can now have sparkling water on hand whenever you want, and it won't break the bank. One SodaStream CO2 refill cartridge makes sixty liters of water which means each liter is priced at less than fifty cents. Once you see how much money you can save using your SodaStream, you will never want to pay for pre-made sparkling water ever again.

Use Fruit Juices and Other Natural Flavors

Since you control all of the flavors that you use with your SodaStream, you can get really creative when it comes to making your own drinks. In our recipes section, we will cover over a hundred ways that you can make new and exciting drinks using fruit juices and other natural flavors. We will show you how to make syrups and extract that you can concentrate in order to give your SodaStream water a robust kick of flavor that will rival or exceed any store bought soda on the market. And because you are in total control over everything that you use, you never have to worry about the ingredients you are drinking.

Use Less Sugar Than Pre-Made Soda

One of the biggest concerns with soda these days is the amount of sugar they contain. We've all heard that too much sugar is a leading cause of many different illnesses, and luckily, your SodaStream can help you make refreshing beverages using less sugar than conventional sodas. We're going to cover how to make syrups using fruits and berries, but we're also going to cover the wide array of flavors that are currently available that taste great but contain far less sugar. SodaStream even makes their own flavor syrups, many of which contain no sugar at all. They are also not made with aspartame, an artificial sweetener that has also been linked to health issue.

The Benefits of Using Filtered Water

Whether you are carbonating your water or drinking it still, the benefits of using filtered water are many. In many parts of the country, tap water still contains levels of chemicals that are not safe for consumption. For the healthiest results, we suggest investing in a simple water filtering system that will remove many of these harmful chemicals while still preserving vital minerals found in water. When coupled with your SodaStream, a water filtering system will result in crisper, cleaner, better tasting sparkling water and flavored beverages.

CHAPTER 3: A BRIEF HISTORY OF SODA DRINKS

The Science of Carbonation

Believe it or not, carbonated beverages have been around longer than we have. Our first encounters with sparkling water came from naturally occurring springs located all over the world, and as soon as people discovered that sparkling water came right out of the ground, it was considered a luxury product. As time went on, however, scientists realized that they could replicate this natural phenomenon and provide many more people with this refreshing treat. As early as the late 1700s, scientists at the Schweppes company were figuring out ways to artificially add carbon dioxide to water to simulate natural spring water.

The Introduction of New Flavors

After we discovered how to add carbon dioxide to water, it was only a matter of time before we started adding flavors to it. The first documented case of a flavored sparkling beverage was in the early 1800s when the first sparkling ginger beer was invented. It bore the name beer because at that point beer and champagne were the only flavored sparkling beverages that anyone drank. It wasn't long, however, until soda makers started experimenting with other flavors. Since fruits and berries didn't keep as long, the earliest, and still favorite, soda flavors were made from things that didn't spoil so easily. Believe it or not, tree bark was one of the first things used to flavor sodas and we still enjoy these flavors today when we drink root beer and birch beer. The real soda revolution happened when a chemist in Atlanta Georgia made an extract from an exotic nut and gave the world Coca Cola.

How Coca Cola Changed the World

In 1886, a chemist named John Pemberton invented a sparkling beverage made with an extract from the cola nut that he calls Coca Cola. This was partly because at the time, Coca Cola also contained an extract from the coca leaf: cocaine. It wasn't long, however, before Pemberton was convinced to remove the cocaine, but the name stuck. When the Coca Cola company incorporated several years later, the true revolution happened. The company realized that transporting liquid was too costly to make a large profit, so they decided to try something new. Instead of making all of the soda themselves, they just made the syrup. They then set up bottling plants all over the United States and sent the syrup to the bottlers to make their own soda. This meant that the soda didn't have to travel great distances to consumers, and Coca Cola could still make sure that a Coke tasted the same no matter where you bought it. The original formula is still a highly guarded secret and only a few people in the world know what it is. The formula is kept in a vault near Atlanta Georgia.

The Future of Soda

With growing concerns about the health effects of soda, one thing is for sure: We won't be drinking soda the same way for much longer. We have become aware of the health risks that soda causes, but that doesn't mean that people don't still want delicious carbonated beverages. The SodaStream is part of the next chapter in soda making. Because the SodaStream allows you to control exactly what goes into your soda, you can avoid the harmful ingredients that can cause illness. We are also seeing a new crop of bottled soda that uses natural ingredients and less harmful sweeteners, and now you can make these drinks at home, any time you want.

CHAPTER 4: HOW TO USE YOUR SODA MAKER

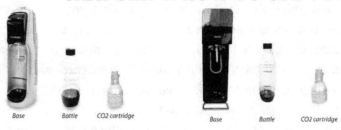

How to Set up Your SodaStream in Minutes

The great thing about the SodaStream is how easy it is to use. And part of its ease of use comes from the fact that setting it up really couldn't be simpler. The SodaStream comes in three basic pieces. The base, the bottles, and the CO2 cartridge. No batteries or electricity is required, so feel free to use your SodaStream wherever you want. Simply open the back compartment on the base, remove the safety cap from the CO2 cartridge, and insert the cartridge into the base. Close the back of the base and you are now ready to start making your own sodas.

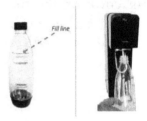

How to Make The Perfect Sparkling Water

The first step in using your SodaStream is to make sparkling water. You will end up doing this step first for almost all of the drinks you will ever make. Start by filling a SodaStream bottle with tap or filtered water. Each bottle has a maximum fill line and to avoid overflow it is very important that you fill the bottles exactly to this line. Then, simply screw the bottle into the base of the machine. When you are ready to carbonate, gently press the top of the SodaStream and you will notice the CO2 rushing into the water. Once you have reached your desired carbonation level, just unscrew the bottle. Now you have a liter of freshly carbonated water that you can drink as is, or add flavors to it.

How to Use Flavors to Make Sweet Sodas

In our recipes section, we will cover many different ideas for how to create interesting beverages that will delight your friends and family. We will teach you how to make familiar flavors as well as new ideas that you may never have considered.

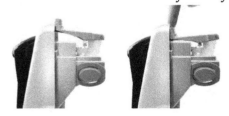

How to Control Your Carbonation Level

Since the SodaStream allows you to customize the amount of carbonation you add to your sparkling water, you will need to know how to get just the right amount. This will require a certain amount of experimentation as different people have different preferences when it comes to carbonation levels. The SodaStream has three basic options for different carbonation. The first is the lowest level, and is best if you prefer the taste and feel of natural sparkling spring water. Since natural spring water tends to be less carbonated than artificially made sparkling water, this setting will work best for that. The medium level will most closely resemble store bought sodas. The highest level is for people who really enjoy a powerful kick of carbonation.

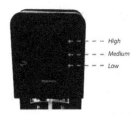

In order to achieve these different levels, you will need to push down on the top of the SodaStream for different periods of time. Once the desired level is reached, simply stop pressing. Carefully unscrew the bottle and you have a perfect liter of water.

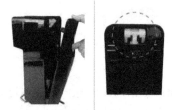

The Best Way to Clean and Store Your SodaStream and Bottles

The SodaStream is extremely easy to use, but it's also very easy to clean. For the base of the unit, you will only ever need to wipe it down with a wet towel. The bottles are not recommended for dishwasher use, because dishwashers can harm the integrity of the plastic and lead to bottles that don't hold carbonation as well. It is recommended that you rinse the bottles with soap and water and allow to dry. The SodaStream is an attractive item to display on your counter, but you can also keep in in a cabinet when it is not in use.

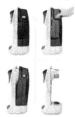

CHAPTER 5: PRO TIPS

What is The Best Amount of Flavoring to Use?

Much like your desired level of carbonation, the amount of flavoring is entirely up to you. Some people prefer very strongly flavored sodas, while others prefer something more subtle. If you are using flavors pre-made by SodaStream, you will find that each one has individual recommendations for how many drops of flavoring are encouraged for a liter of water. Of course, these are merely recommendations, and you will surely find your own optimum level of flavor. To start, we encourage you to start with a small amount of flavor, then have a taste. If it needs a little more, add more and taste again. In no time you will become an expert at knowing just how much you need.

How to Avoid Overflowing Your SodaStream

Since no one wants carbonated liquids spraying all over their kitchen, it is important to follow a couple of simply guidelines for how to avoid this. You might be tempted to flavor some water first and then carbonate it. This is a mistake because all soda making systems are only designed to carbonate plain water. Even soda fountains work on this principle. The water is carbonated and then as it is being dispensed, the flavor is added to it. Because adding flavors beforehand will change the density of the water, the result is that the carbonation will make the bottle overflow once it is removed from the machine. This also applies to things like juice.

How to Make Sparkling Wine with The SodaStream

While we do not recommend that you carbonate water that has already been flavored, there is a method to turn regular wine into sparkling wine. It should be noted that this pro tip should only be used with white wine. You should use the driest white wine you can find because drier wines contain less sugar and are therefore easier to carbonate. First, start by filling the bottle only halfway with wine. Attach it to the machine and gently press for just a couple of seconds. This should be less carbonation than you will need to even reach the first carbonation level. Slowly unscrew the bottle allowing it to release CO2 very slowly. Give it a taste to see if it has enough carbonation and if not, repeat that process until it does. When carbonating wine, it is important to clean your SodaStream right after you are finished.

Make Your Own Syrups for The SodaStream

In our recipes section, we will go into greater depth about how to make custom flavors to use with your SodaStream, but the world of possibilities is almost limitless. From fruit and berry syrups and extracts, to more savory things like chocolate and nut flavors, you can have fun trying new ideas to make unique and delicious sodas for any occasion. We will also teach you how to make low sugar syrups and flavors that require no added sugar at all.

Make Name Brand Sodas with Your SodaStream

Believe it or not, you can buy some of your favorite soda flavors and add them to water you carbonate yourself at home. Many large brands actually sell bottles of their concentrated syrups that can be added directly to your sparkling water to create exact replicas of your favorite name brand sodas. You may need to do a little experimentation to get the flavor level just right, but the money you will save making these sodas at home will make it well worth it. To find these syrups contact your local cash and carry stores or restaurant supply stores. You will be able to buy enough syrup to make soda for a very long time, and will cost a tiny fraction of pre-made sodas.

CHAPTER 6: MIXED FRUIT SODAS

Apple Cinnamon Soda

SERVINGS: 8 | PREP TIME: 5 MINUTES | COOK TIME: 20 MINUTES

This sweet spiced soda is perfect for Fall with its crisp apple flavor and the addition of natural cinnamon. For best results use fresh pressed apple cider.

INGREDIENTS:

2 cups apple cider

1/2 cup sugar

2 whole cinnamon sticks

2 liters SodaStream sparkling water

INSTRUCTIONS:

1. In a medium sauce pan, combine the apple cider, sugar, and cinnamon sticks. Bring to a boil and then reduce heat to a simmer. Cook until the mixture has reduced by half and the sugar is dissolved completely.
2. Remove from heat and remove the cinnamon sticks from the cider. Allow to cool completely.
3. Use your SodaStream to carbonate 2 liters of cold water.
4. Fill glasses with ice and add 3 tablespoons of the apple syrup to each glass. Then fill with SodaStream water.

Apple Pomegranate Soda

SERVINGS: 4 | PREP TIME: 10 MINUTES | COOK TIME: 30 MINUTES

This sweet and tart fruit soda combines the complimentary flavors of apple and pomegranate for a unique blend that is further enhanced by a splash of effervescence.

INGREDIENTS:

1 cup apple cider (preferably fresh pressed)

1/2 cup pomegranate juice

1 cup sugar

1 liter SodaStream sparkling water

Ice

INSTRUCTIONS:

1. In a medium sauce pan, combine the apple cider, pomegranate juice, and sugar. Bring to a boil and then lower to a simmer.
2. Cook the juice mixture until it has reduced and is beginning to thicken.
3. Remove from heat and let cool completely. Chill in the fridge until cold. Use your SodaStream to carbonate 1 liter of cold water.
4. Fill glasses with ice and add 4 tablespoons of the syrup to each glass. Fill the glass with SodaStream water and serve.

Banana Soda

SERVINGS: 10 | PREP TIME: 15 MINUTES | COOK TIME: 15 MINUTES

This unusual fruit soda uses natural banana flavor for a refreshing tropical flavor that will be sure to delight your friends and family on a hot summer day.

INGREDIENTS:

1 teaspoon banana flavor

1 pound white sugar

1 cup water

2 tablespoons lemon juice

2 liters SodaStream sparkling water

INSTRUCTIONS:

1. In a pot, combine the water and white sugar. Heat to a boil and stir until the sugar is completely dissolved. Remove from heat and allow to cool completely.

2. Once the syrup is completely cool, add the banana flavor and lemon juice. Use your SodaStream to carbonate 2 liters of cold water.

3. Add 2 tablespoons of syrup to each glass and top with sparkling water. Add some ice and serve.

Cantaloupe Float

SERVINGS: 4 | PREP TIME: 10 MINUTES | COOK TIME: 10 MINUTES

This delicious melon smoothie soda is perfectly refreshing on its own, but the addition of a scoop of vanilla ice cream will turn a light, fresh beverage into a fun dessert in seconds.

INGREDIENTS:

1 cantaloupe

1/3 cup sugar

1/3 cup water

1 liter SodaStream sparkling water

1 cup vanilla ice cream

INSTRUCTIONS:

1. Cut melon in half and remove the flesh, cutting it into chunks. Place 1 cup of the chunks in the freezer and allow to completely freeze. Put the other chunks of cantaloupe in the refrigerator.

2. In a small sauce pan, combine the sugar and water and heat over medium heat until the sugar has completely dissolved. Remove from heat and allow to cool.

3. Place the unfrozen cantaloupe into a blender and blend until pureed.

4. Use your SodaStream to carbonate 1 liter of cold water.

5. Add 1 cup of SodaStream water to the cantaloupe puree and stir.

6. Remove the frozen cantaloupe from the freezer and add the cubes to glasses, then pour in the cantaloupe soda and top with a scoop of vanilla ice cream.

Concord Grape and Lemon Soda

SERVINGS: 6 | PREP TIME: 20 MINUTES | COOK TIME: 10 MINUTES

This delightful fruit flavored soda is a refreshing way to use Concord grapes to make an interesting and flavorful beverage. The addition of lemons and cinnamon combine for a complex flavor that doesn't require using a great deal of added sugar.

INGREDIENTS:

2 lemons

1 pound concord grapes

1/2 cup white sugar

1 cinnamon stick

2 tablespoons still water

1 liter SodaStream sparkling water

INSTRUCTIONS:

1. Zest the lemons and combine the zest with the grapes, sugar, and cinnamon with the still water in a large saucepan. Cook on low until the sugar has dissolved and then simmer for another 20 minutes until the grapes have a jam-like consistency.

2. Let the mixture cool and then strain the liquid and discard the grape skins and cinnamon.

3. Juice the lemons used for zest.

4. Use your SodaStream to carbonate one liter of cold water.

5. Fill six glasses with ice and add two teaspoons of lemon juice and two tablespoons of the grape syrup to each glass.

6. Top each glass with SodaStream Sparkling water and serve.

Homemade Grape Soda

SERVINGS: 4 | PREP TIME: 10 MINUTES | COOK TIME: 30 MINUTES

Grape soda has been around for nearly a century, and now you can make your own grape soda at home using fresh grapes instead of artificial flavors. You can use any type of grapes you'd like, but we recommend using seedless black grapes for the best balance of flavor and color.

INGREDIENTS:

1 pound fresh grapes

1/2 cup still water

Juice of 1/2 lemon

1 liter SodaStream sparkling water

INSTRUCTIONS:

1. In a large pot combine the grapes, still water, and lemon juice over medium heat. Simmer until the grapes are very soft. This should take about 20 minutes. As the grapes cook, smash them with a wooden spoon.
2. Pour the mixture into a blender or food processor and blend until smooth. Strain the mixture and discard the solids.
3. Place the grape syrup into the refrigerator until it is chilled. Use your SodaStream to carbonate 1 liter of cold water.
4. Fill glasses with ice, and the fill the glasses halfway with syrup and then top with SodaStream water.

Italian Black Cherry Cream Soda

SERVINGS: 4 | PREP TIME: 5 MINUTES | COOK TIME: 5 MINUTES

This rich creamy traditional Italian soda can be made with a number of different syrups, but this recipe features black cherry syrup for a sweet and tart soda that is creamy and satisfying.

INGREDIENTS:

12 tablespoons Italian black cherry syrup

4 tablespoons half and half

Ice

1 liter SodaStream sparkling water

Whipped cream (optional)

INSTRUCTIONS:

1. Use your SodaStream to carbonate 1 liter of cold water.
2. Fill 4 glasses with ice and add 3 tablespoons of black cherry syrup to each glass.
3. Fill the glasses to the top with SodaStream sparkling water and add one tablespoon of half and half to each glass. Top with whipped cream and serve immediately.

Maple Cherry Cream Soda

SERVINGS: 8 | PREP TIME: 10 MINUTES | COOK TIME: 20 MINUTES

This take on an Italian soda has multiple layers of flavors thanks to the earthy, sweet maple syrup as well as fresh sweet cherries. The addition of a hint of cream makes for a soda that is refreshing and smooth.

INGREDIENTS:

1-1/2 pounds fresh cherries, pitted

1 cup still water

3/4 cups sugar

1/4 cup real maple syrup

1 teaspoon vanilla extract

8 tablespoons half and half

2 liters SodaStream sparkling water

INSTRUCTIONS:

1. In a medium sauce pan, combine the cherries, still water, sugar, maple syrup, and vanilla extract over medium heat. Stir until all of the sugar has dissolved and simmer for another 15 minutes. Remove from heat, strain, and allow to cool to room temperature.
2. Use your SodaStream to carbonate 2 liters of cold water.
3. Fill glasses with ice and add 3 tablespoons of the cherry syrup and top with SodaStream water. Then add one tablespoon of half and half to each glass and stir.

Maple Peach Soda

This soda uses real maple syrup as its base, but the addition of ripe white peaches makes for an interesting combination of flavors that complement and enhance each other.

INGREDIENTS:

1/2 cup real maple syrup

1/4 cup water

2 cups ripe white peaches, chopped

1 liter SodaStream sparkling water

INSTRUCTIONS:

1. In a medium sauce pan, combine the maple syrup, water, and peaches. Heat until the peaches begin to soften. Remove from heat.
2. Pour the maple peach mixture into a blender and puree. Then allow to cool completely.
3. Use your SodaStream to carbonate 1 liter of cold water.
4. Fill 4 glasses with ice and add 1/3 cup of the peach puree to each glass. Then add 1 cup of SodaStream water. Stir and serve immediately.

Sour Cherry Soda

SERVINGS: 8 | PREP TIME: 10 MINUTES | COOK TIME: 30 MINUTES

This all natural take on an old fashioned soda fountain favorite uses fresh cherries and tart lemon juice to create a syrup that is robust and flavorful for any occasion.

INGREDIENTS:

1 pound fresh sour cherries, pitted

2 cups sugar

juice from 1/2 lemon

2 liters SodaStream sparkling water

INSTRUCTIONS:

1. In a medium sauce pan, combine the cherries, sugar, and lemon juice and bring to a gentle boil. Simmer for about 30 minutes or until the cherries have broken down.
2. Remove from heat and strain out all of the solids from the syrup and discard. Then allow the syrup to cool completely before using.
3. Use your SodaStream to carbonate 2 liters of cold water.
4. Fill glasses with ice and pour in 1/4 cup of the cherry syrup into each glass. Top with SodaStream water and serve.

Summertime Peach Soda

SERVINGS: 4-6 | PREP TIME: 10 MINUTES | COOK TIME: 20 MINUTES

This refreshing peach soda relies on ripe summer peaches for a punch of flavor that you could never get with store bought soda. The complex flavors enhance the natural sweetness of the peach for a robust drink that you can enjoy as long as fresh peaches are available.

INGREDIENTS:

1-1/2 pounds peaches that are very ripe, peeled and sliced

1 tablespoon fresh lemon juice

1/4 teaspoon salt

1 cup still water

1/2 cup sugar

1 liter SodaStream sparkling water

INSTRUCTIONS:

1. Peel and slice the peaches and remove the pit. Then mix them in a large bowl with the lemon juice and salt.
2. In a medium sauce pan, heat the still water almost to a boil, remove from heat and stir in the sugar until it has dissolved completely.
3. Add the peaches to the bowl with the sugar water and let stand for 10 minutes.
4. In a blender, puree the peach and sugar water mixture, then strain out the solids with a mesh strainer. Place in the refrigerator and chill.
5. Use your SodaStream to carbonate 1 liter of cold water.
6. Fill glasses with ice and add 1/2 cup of the peach syrup to each glass and top with SodaStream water.

Peach and Thyme Soda

SERVINGS: 4 | PREP TIME: 5 MINUTES | COOK TIME: 30 MINUTES

This naturally flavored fruit soda combines the mellow sweetness of fresh peached with the earthy aroma of fresh thyme leaves for a complex and refreshing beverage.

INGREDIENTS:

3 large peaches, pitted and sliced

1/2 cup sugar

4 sprigs thyme

1 liter SodaStream sparkling water

INSTRUCTIONS:

1. In a large sauce pan, combine the peaches, sugar, and thyme. Smash the peaches with a spoon and cook for about 30 minutes or until the peaches have completely broken down.
2. Strain the mixture through a sieve and discard the solids. Allow the syrup to cool completely before using.
3. Use your SodaStream to carbonate one liter of cold water.
4. Add ice to four glasses and pour 1/4 cup of the syrup into each glass. Fill with SodaStream sparkling water and serve.

Pomegranate Rosewater Soda

SERVINGS: 2 | PREP TIME: 1 MINUTE | COOK TIME: 1 MINUTE

The great thing about pomegranate juice is that it's so flavorful on its own that you don't need to make a concentrated syrup in order to enjoy a full flavored soda. The addition of rosewater to this soda adds a nice floral undertone to the robust flavor of pomegranate.

INGREDIENTS:

1 cup pomegranate juice

1/2 teaspoon rosewater

2 teaspoons lime juice

1 liter SodaStream sparkling water

INSTRUCTIONS:

1. Use your SodaStream to carbonate 1 liter of cold water.
2. Fill 2 glasses with ice and add 1/2 cup pomegranate juice, 1/4 teaspoon rosewater, and 1 teaspoon of lime juice to each glass.
3. Then fill with SodaStream water and stir.

Watermelon Peach Lime Soda

SERVINGS: 4 | PREP TIME: 5 MINUTES | COOK TIME: 20 MINUTES

This light and refreshing soda combines fresh watermelon, peach, and lime for a subtle yet tart soda that is perfect for hot summer days. It can also be made into a sparkling cocktail by adding a shot of chilled vodka.

INGREDIENTS:

1 ripe peach, peeled and sliced

2 cups watermelon, cubed

Juice of 2 limes

1/2 cup still water

1/2 cup sugar

1 liter SodaStream sparkling water

INSTRUCTIONS:

1. In a small sauce pan, combine the still water and sugar over medium heat. Stir until all of the sugar has dissolved. Remove from heat and add the lime juice. Allow to cool completely.
2. In a blender or food processor, combine the peach and watermelon. Blend until smooth.
3. Use your SodaStream to carbonate 1 liter of cold water.
4. Fill glasses with ice and add 2 tablespoons of the peach-watermelon puree and 2 tablespoons of the lime syrup.
5. Top with SodaStream water and stir well.

CHAPTER 7: BERRY SODAS

Blackberry Lime Soda

SERVINGS: 4 | PREP TIME: 5 MINUTES | COOK TIME: 20 MINUTES

This recipe uses fresh blackberries and limes to create a punch of flavor that will invigorate you on a hot summer day. This soda can also be made as a sparkling cocktail by adding a shot of ice cold vodka.

INGREDIENTS:

1 cup fresh blackberries

1 cup still water

3/4 cups sugar

Juice from 1 lime

1 liter SodaStream sparkling water

INSTRUCTIONS:

1. In a medium sauce pan, combine the water, sugar, and blackberries over medium heat and simmer until the blackberries have broken down and become a syrup. This should take about 15 minutes.
2. Remove from heat and strain out all of the solids and stir in the lime juice. Place the syrup in the refrigerator until it is chilled and thickened.
3. Use your SodaStream to carbonate 1 liter of cold water.
4. Fill glasses with ice and add 3 tablespoons of the blackberry syrup to each glass. Top with SodaStream water and stir.

Blackberry Soda

SERVINGS: 8 | PREP TIME: 10 MINUTES | COOK TIME: 25 MINUTES

This soda uses a syrup made from fresh blackberries to make a delicious and refreshing soda that the whole family can enjoy. If you happen to have wild blackberries growing near your house, it's a great way to make the most out of blackberry season.

INGREDIENTS:

1 pint fresh blackberries

1/2 cup sugar

1/2 cup still water

2 tablespoons lemon juice

2 liters SodaStream sparkling water

INSTRUCTIONS:

1. In a medium sauce pan, combine the blackberries, still water, and sugar over medium heat. Cook until the blackberries have broken down, and the sugar is completely dissolved. Remove from heat.
2. Strain out the solids and add the lemon juice to the syrup. Allow to cool completely before using.
3. Use your SodaStream to carbonate 2 liters of cold water.
4. Fill glasses with ice and add 1/4 cup of the blackberry syrup to each glass, then add SodaStream water and stir before servings.

Blueberry Cream Italian Soda

SERVINGS: 8 | PREP TIME: 10 MINUTES | COOK TIME: 15 MINUTES

Italian sodas are great because you can use so many flavors to make so many different drinks. This recipe shows you how to use fresh blueberries to make a syrup that will be the perfect base for Italian sodas.

INGREDIENTS:

1 pound fresh blueberries

1 cup sugar

1 cup still water

3 tablespoons lemon juice

8 tablespoons half and half or heavy cream

2 liters SodaStream sparkling water

INSTRUCTIONS:

1. In a medium sauce pan, combine the blueberries, still water, and sugar. Heat over medium heat and stir until the sugar has dissolved. Then simmer until the blueberries have broken down.
2. Remove from heat and strain the blueberry mixture. Then add the lemon juice and allow to cool completely.
3. Use your SodaStream to carbonate 2 liters of cold water.
4. Fill glasses with ice and add 1/4 cup of the blueberry syrup to each glass.
5. Add one tablespoon of half and half to each glass then fill with SodaStream water.

Blueberry Lemonade Soda

SERVINGS: 6 | PREP TIME: 10 MINUTES | COOK TIME: 30 MINUTES

This sweet and tart take on carbonated lemonade is perfect for entertaining, and you can also experiment with adding a little vodka for a refreshing carbonated cocktail.

INGREDIENTS:

2 cups blueberries

1 cup sugar

1 cup still water

1 cup lemon juice (preferably fresh)

1 liter SodaStream sparkling water

INSTRUCTIONS:

1. In a medium sauce pan, combine the blueberries, sugar, and still water. Heat until the blueberries begin to break down, then simmer an additional 10 minutes, making sure the sugar is completely dissolved.

2. Remove from heat and strain out the solids.

3. When the syrup is cool, add the lemon juice and stir. Carbonate 1 liter of cold water using your SodaStream

4. Add ice to 6 tall glasses and divide the syrup equally among them. Add one cup of SodaStream water to each glass and serve immediately.

Cranberry Soda

SERVINGS: 4 | PREP TIME: 15 MINUTES | COOK TIME: 5 MINUTES

This refreshing tart soda uses natural cranberry juice and is sweetened with honey instead of sugar for a healthier beverage.

INGREDIENTS:

1 cup unsweetened cranberry juice

1 cup honey

1 cup water

1 liter SodaStream sparkling water

INSTRUCTIONS:

1. In a medium sauce pan combine the water and honey over medium heat. Stir until they are blended.
2. Add the cranberry juice and let simmer for about five minutes.
3. Remove from heat and allow to cool completely.
4. Use your SodaStream to carbonate one liter of water on the highest carbonation setting.
5. Fill four glasses with ice and add one quarter of the syrup to each glass, then top with the sparkling water.

Kiwi Strawberry Soda

SERVINGS: 8 | PREP TIME: 10 MINUTES | COOK TIME: 30 MINUTES

Kiwi and strawberry go together so well because the tartness of fresh kiwis and the sweetness of strawberries balance each other perfectly. This recipe shows you how to make a kiwi strawberry syrup that can be the basis for a soda or a sparkling cocktail.

INGREDIENTS:

2 cups fresh strawberries, chopped

2 cups kiwi, peeled and chopped

1/2 cup sugar

1/2 cup still water

2 liters SodaStream sparkling water

INSTRUCTIONS:

1. In a medium sauce pan, combine the strawberries, kiwi, sugar, and still water over medium heat. Cook until the sugar has completely dissolved and the fruit has broken down. Remove from heat.
2. Allow the mixture to steep for 10 minutes and strain out all of the solids, and allow to cool completely.
3. Use your SodaStream to carbonate 2 liters of cold water.
4. Fill glasses with ice and add 1/4 cup of the syrup to each glass. Top with SodaStream water and stir well before serving.

Mulberry Maple Cream Soda

SERVINGS: 8 | PREP TIME: 10 MINUTES | COOK TIME: 20 MINUTES

This creamy Italian style soda uses fresh mulberries along with the flavor of roses to create a sweet and floral drink that is unlike anything you've tasted before. The distinctive flavor of the berries is enhanced by natural maple syrup resulting in a drink that is sure to please everyone.

INGREDIENTS:

1/4 cup rosewater

3 cups mulberries

1 cup sugar

2 tablespoons maple syrup

1 cup still water

1 teaspoon vanilla extract

2 liters SodaStream sparkling water

8 tablespoons half and half

INSTRUCTIONS:

1. In a medium sauce pan, combine the mulberries, sugar, still water, and maple syrup over medium heat. Stir until all of the sugar is dissolved. Remove from heat.
2. Stir in the rosewater and then strain out all of the solids. Allow to cool to room temperature.
3. Use your SodaStream to carbonate 2 liters of cold water.
4. Fill glasses with ice and add 2 tablespoons of the berry syrup and top with SodaStream water. Then add a tablespoon of half and half to each glass before serving.

Raspberry Cream Soda

SERVINGS: 4 | PREP TIME: 5 MINUTES | COOK TIME: 20 MINUTES

You could use store bought syrups to make this rich creamy soda, but we're going to show you how to do it yourself using fresh natural ingredients for a more complex and robust flavor.

INGREDIENTS:

2 cups fresh raspberries

1 whole vanilla bean

2 tablespoons lemon juice

1/2 cup still water

1/2 cup sugar

1 liter SodaStream sparkling water

INSTRUCTIONS:

1. In a medium sauce pan, combine the raspberries, vanilla bean, still water, and sugar over medium heat. Stir until the sugar has dissolved and the raspberries have broken down. It should take about 15 minutes.

2. Remove from heat and strain out the solids. Then add the lemon juice and allow the syrup to cool completely before using.

3. Use your SodaStream to carbonate 1 liter of cold water. Fill 4 glasses with ice and pour in 1/4 cup of the raspberry vanilla syrup to each glass. Fill with SodaStream water and serve.

Raspberry Ginger Soda

SERVINGS: 4 | PREP TIME: 5 MINUTES | COOK TIME: 30 MINUTES

Fresh ginger was one of the first ingredients ever used in soda making and it is still popular today because it contains just the right amount of sweetness and spiciness to create a beverage that is full of complexity. This soda pairs fresh ginger with fresh raspberries for a fruity and spicy soda that is sure to delight everyone.

INGREDIENTS:

4 cups fresh raspberries

1 cup still water

1 cup sugar

4 tablespoons lemon or lime juice

1/4 cup fresh ginger, peeled and sliced

1 liter SodaStream sparkling water

INSTRUCTIONS:

1. In a medium sauce pan, combine the still water, sugar, and ginger over medium heat. Stir until all of the sugar has dissolved and then add the raspberries. Simmer until the raspberries have broken down, about 15 minutes.

2. Remove from heat and strain out all of the solids. Allow the syrup to cool completely before using.

3. Use your SodaStream to carbonate 1 liter of cold water.

4. Fill 4 glasses with ice and add 1/4 cup of the raspberry ginger syrup to each glass. Fill with SodaStream water and serve.

Raspberry Key Lime Soda

SERVINGS: 6 | PREP TIME: 5 MINUTES | COOK TIME: 15 MINUTES

The combination of raspberries and sweet key lime juice is excellent when combined with sparkling water from your soda stream. You can even decide how strong you want your flavor to be by adding as much syrup as you want. You can either make a full flavored soda, or a subtle flavored sparkling water.

INGREDIENTS:

1 pound fresh raspberries

1 cup sugar

Zest from 2 key limes

Juice from 2 key limes

1/3 cup still water

1 liter SodaStream sparkling water

INSTRUCTIONS:

1. In a medium sauce pan, combine the raspberries and sugar over medium heat.
2. Zest and juice the limes and add the zest to the raspberries. Mash the berries well with a spoon and continue to cook for several minutes.
3. Add the still water and simmer another 5 minutes.
4. Strain out the solids and add the lime juice to the syrup. Allow to cool completely.
5. Fill 6 glasses with ice and add 2 tablespoons of syrup to each glass. Top with SodaStream water and serve immediately.

Raspberry Vanilla Soda

SERVINGS: 8 | PREP TIME: 25 MINUTES | COOK TIME: 10 MINUTES

The complex berry soda is perfect for entertaining or just enjoying on a hot summer day. The mix of fresh raspberries and vanilla produces a fruity yet creamy flavor that is sure to be enjoyed by all.

INGREDIENTS:

8 ounces fresh raspberries

1/2 cup sugar

1 cup still water

2 tablespoons lime juice

1 teaspoon vanilla extract

2 liters SodaStream sparkling water

Mint leaves for garnish (optional)

INSTRUCTIONS:

1. In a medium sauce pan combine the raspberries, sugar, still water, lime juice, and vanilla extract over medium heat.
2. Heat for about 20 minutes or until the raspberries have broken down. Remove from heat.
3. When the mixture has cooled, strain it through a mesh strainer to eliminate the seeds and pulp.
4. Use your SodaStream to carbonate 2 liters of cold water.
5. Fill glasses with ice, and add two tablespoons of the raspberry syrup to each glass. Fill with SodaStream water and garnish with a mint leaf.

Strawberry Basil Soda

SERVINGS: 4 | PREP TIME: 10 MINUTES | COOK TIME: 15 MINUTES

The sweetness of strawberries is enhanced by the addition of earthy basil for a soda that is well balanced and refreshing. Try to use ripe strawberries in season for the most flavorful soda possible.

INGREDIENTS:

1 pound fresh strawberries

Juice of 1 lemon

1/2 cup basil leaves

1 cup sugar

1 liter SodaStream sparkling water

INSTRUCTIONS:

1. Place the strawberries in a blender and blend until smooth. Strain the puree and discard the solids.

2. In a medium sauce pan, combine the strawberry juice, lemon juice, basil, and sugar over medium heat. Stir until all of the sugar has dissolved and remove from heat. Strain once again to remove the solids, and allow to cool completely.

3. Use your SodaStream to carbonate 1 liter of cold water.

4. Fill 4 glasses with ice and add 2 tablespoons of the syrup to each glass, and top with SodaStream water. If this is not flavorful enough, feel free to add more syrup until you have reached your desired flavor level.

Strawberry Black Pepper Soda

SERVINGS: 8 | PREP TIME: 24 HOURS | COOK TIME: 10 MINUTES

This soda combines the sweet flavor of fresh strawberries with the spicy, earthy flavor of black pepper for an interesting and refreshing beverage. The longer you allow the pepper to infuse into the syrup the stronger the flavor will become.

INGREDIENTS:

2 pounds fresh strawberries, sliced

3-1/2 cups sugar

3 tablespoons fresh orange juice

2 tablespoons crushed black peppercorns

SodaStream sparkling water

INSTRUCTIONS:

1. In a large bowl, combine the strawberries and 2 cups of sugar. Stir well so that all of the strawberries are coated in sugar. Then cover the mixture with the remaining 1 1/2 cups of sugar.
2. Allow the berries to macerate for 12 hours, stirring occasionally.
3. Once the strawberries have macerated, strain out the liquid and discard the solids.
4. Stir in the orange juice and peppercorns and pour into a glass jar. Allow the syrup to steep for at least 12 hours.
5. Use your SodaStream to carbonate 1 liter of cold water. Fill glasses with ice and add 2 tablespoons of the syrup to each glass. Top with SodaStream water and serve.

Strawberry Pineapple Soda

SERVINGS: 3 | PREP TIME: 10 MINUTES | COOK TIME: 10 MINUTES

This tropical treat is perfect for kicking back on a summer day and it's also a great way to put that ripe pineapple to good use. Another great feature of this soda is that it relies mostly on the natural sweetness of the fruits and only uses a small amount of added sugar.

INGREDIENTS:

1 pint fresh strawberries, chopped

1 cup pineapple juice

1 tablespoon sugar

1 liter SodaStream sparkling water

INSTRUCTIONS:

1. In a small bowl, combine the strawberries and sugar and allow to sit for about 10 minutes, or until the strawberries start to break down.
2. In a blender or food processor, combine the strawberries with the pineapple juice and add the sugar. Puree until the mixtures is smooth. Strain the mixture to remove all of the seeds and other solids.
3. Use your SodaStream to carbonate 1 liter of cold water.
4. Fill glasses with ice and pour in 2/3 of a cup of the puree and top with SodaStream water.
5. Stir well and serve immediately.

Strawberry Rosewater Soda

SERVINGS: 4 | PREP TIME: 10 MINUTES | COOK TIME: 30 MINUTES

The sweetness of fresh strawberries is complimented by the subtle floral flavor of rosewater for an unexpected and refreshing soda that balances just the right amount of sweetness with the complex flavors of roses.

INGREDIENTS:

1 pound fresh strawberries, sliced

1/3 cup rosewater

1/4 cup still water

1/2 cup sugar

1 liter SodaStream sparkling water

INSTRUCTIONS:

1. In a medium sauce pan, combine the strawberries, rosewater, still water, and sugar, over medium heat until the sugar has completely dissolved. Lower the heat and allow to simmer for about 15 minutes.
2. Transfer the mixture to a blender or food processor and blend until the mixture is smooth. Strain out all of the solids and allow the syrup to cool completely.
3. Use your SodaStream to carbonate 1 liter of cold water.
4. Fill 4 glasses with ice and pour in 1/3 cup of the strawberry syrup, and top with SodaStream water.

Strawberry Soda

SERVINGS: 10 | PREP TIME: 20 MINUTES | COOK TIME: 10 MINUTES

This fun refreshing berry soda is great for a hot summer day, and because it uses fresh strawberries you will be getting a full day's dose of vitamin C with every glass you drink. You can even limit the processed sugar by substituting agave syrup.

INGREDIENTS:

1 pound fresh strawberries, sliced

1 cup sugar or agave syrup

1/2 cup water

2 tablespoons lemon juice

3 liters SodaStream sparkling water

INSTRUCTIONS:

1. In a large bowl combine the sliced strawberries and half of the sugar. Mix well and allow to macerate until the strawberries become mushy.

2. In a large pot, combine the macerated strawberries, lemon juice, water, and remaining sugar. Heat over low heat until the mixture simmers and the sugar dissolves.

3. Allow the mixture to cool completely and strain through a mesh strainer, discarding the solids.

4. Use your SodaStream to carbonate water. Then add four to six tablespoons of syrup to each liter.

Strawberry Tarragon Soda

SERVINGS: 8 | PREP TIME: 24 HOURS | COOK TIME: 1 HOUR

This soda takes a little longer to make but the result is totally worth it. The flavor combination of the strawberries and tarragon takes a while to develop but once it has, you will have created a soda that is rich in flavor and complexity. Try adding a shot of tequila to the soda for a delicious sparkling cocktail.

INGREDIENTS:

1 cup fresh strawberries, sliced

1/4 cup sugar

4 sprigs fresh tarragon

3/4 cups white wine vinegar

2 liters SodaStream sparkling water

INSTRUCTIONS:

1. Place the strawberries and sugar in a bowl and allow them to macerate for 2 hours. Stir every once in a while.
2. In a jar, combine the vinegar and tarragon. Seal and allow to sit at room temperature.
3. Once the strawberries have been sitting for 2 hours, strain out the solids, and add the juice to the jar with the vinegar and tarragon. Place in the refrigerator overnight to develop flavor.
4. Use your SodaStream to carbonate some cold water. Fill glasses with ice and add 2 tablespoons of the strawberry tarragon syrup, and top with SodaStream water.

Strawberry Vanilla Soda

SERVINGS: 4 | PREP TIME: 10 MINUTES | COOK TIME: 20 MINUTES

This soda uses the natural flavors of vanilla extract and fresh strawberries to create a creamy tasting soda without using any cream.

INGREDIENTS:

1 pint fresh strawberries, sliced

2 teaspoons vanilla extract

1/2 cup sugar

1/2 cup still water

1 liter SodaStream sparkling water

INSTRUCTIONS:

1. In a medium sauce pan, combine the strawberries, vanilla extract, still water, and sugar over medium heat. Cook until the strawberries have broken down and the sugar is completely dissolved.
2. Remove from heat and strain out the solids.
3. Then allow to cool completely.
4. Use your SodaStream to carbonate 1 liter of cold water.
5. Fill 4 glasses with ice and pour in 1/3 cup of the syrup, and top with SodaStream water.

CHAPTER 8: CITRUS SODAS

Blood Orange Soda

SERVINGS: 6 | PREP TIME: 10 MINUTES | COOK TIME: 10 MINUTES

Blood oranges are only in season for a short time each year, so try to find as many uses for them as possible before they disappear. This refreshing simple soda uses the juice as well as the peels of the blood orange to balance sweet and sour.

INGREDIENTS:

1 cup water

1/2 cup sugar

Skins and juice from 3 blood oranges

1 liter SodaStream sparkling water

INSTRUCTIONS:

1. In a medium sauce pan, combine the water and sugar and orange skins. Heat over medium heat until the sugar has completely dissolved.
2. Remove from heat and add the orange juice. Allow the mixture to cool completely.
3. Once it is cool, remove the skins from the mixture.
4. Use your SodaStream to carbonate one liter of water. Use the setting that will provide the highest carbonation.
5. Add ice, and 2-4 tablespoons of the syrup to each glass depending on how strong you want the soda to be, and top with SodaStream water.

Cherry Limeade Soda

SERVINGS: 4 | PREP TIME: 10 MINUTES | COOK TIME: 25 MINUTES

The classic combination of cherry and lime never disappoints. This recipe lets you use your SodaStream to make this delicious flavor combination into a robust and refreshing soda.

INGREDIENTS:

2/3 cups sugar

2/3 cups still water

1/2 cup lime juice

1-1/2 cups unsweetened cherry juice

1 liter SodaStream sparkling water

INSTRUCTIONS:

1. In a medium sauce pan, combine the still water and sugar over medium heat. Stir until the sugar has dissolved. Remove from heat and allow to cool completely.
2. Juice the limes, and once the syrup has cooled, combine the syrup, lime juice, and cherry juice.
3. Use your SodaStream to carbonate 1 liter of cold water.
4. Fill glasses with ice and fill halfway with the cherry lime syrup, and top with SodaStream water. Stir and serve immediately.

Classic Lemon Italian Soda

SERVINGS: 4 | PREP TIME: 5 MINUTES | COOK TIME: 20 MINUTES

This tart lemon soda is simple and refreshing because it uses natural lemon juice for a clean, crisp taste.

INGREDIENTS:

1 cup sugar

1 cup still water

Juice from 4 lemons

1 liter SodaStream sparkling water

INSTRUCTIONS:

1. In a medium sauce pan, combine the still water and sugar over medium heat. Stir until all of the sugar has dissolved. Remove from heat and add the lemon juice. Allow to cool completely.
2. Use your SodaStream to carbonate 1 liter of cold water.
3. Fill glasses with ice and add 3 tablespoons of the lemon syrup. Top with SodaStream water and stir.

Clementine Pomegranate Soda

SERVINGS: 4 | PREP TIME: 10 MINUTES | COOK TIME: 10 MINUTES

Clementines are only in season for a short time each year, and their juice is perfect for making flavorful sodas that the whole family will enjoy. This soda combines fresh clementine juice with robust pomegranate juice for a truly unforgettable soda. Once you've had a sip of this, you'll wish that Clementines were available all year round.

INGREDIENTS:

1 cup clementine juice

1/2 cup pomegranate juice

1/2 cup sugar

1/2 cup still water

1 liter SodaStream sparkling water

INSTRUCTIONS:

1. In a medium sauce pan, combine the still water and sugar over medium heat, and cook until the sugar has completely dissolved.
2. Add the Clementine juice and pomegranate juice and simmer until the mixture has a syrupy consistency. This should take about 10 minutes. Remove from heat and allow to cool completely before using.
3. Use your SodaStream to carbonate 1 liter of cold water.
4. Fill 4 glasses with ice and pour 1/3 cup of the syrup into each glass. Top with SodaStream water and stir before serving.

Coconut Lime Soda

SERVINGS: 4 | PREP TIME: 10 MINUTES | COOK TIME: 20 MINUTES

This tropical treat uses coconut syrup and homemade lime syrup to pack a flavorful punch with the mellow flavor of coconut to soften the tartness of the lime. You can also make this into a fun cocktail with the addition of 1 1/2 ounces of rum.

INGREDIENTS:

1 cup still water

1 cup sugar

Juice from 4 limes

Zest from 4 limes

4 tablespoons coconut syrup

1 liter SodaStream sparkling water

INSTRUCTIONS:

1. In a medium sauce pan, combine the still water and sugar. Heat to a gentle boil and cook until the sugar has completely dissolved. Remove from heat.
2. Add the lime juice and zest to the syrup and allow to steep for 10 minutes.
3. Use a strainer to strain out the zest, then allow the syrup to cool completely.
4. Use your SodaStream to carbonate 1 liter of cold water.
5. Fill 4 glasses with ice and add 1/2 cup lime syrup and 1 tablespoon coconut syrup to each glass. Then fill with SodaStream water and stir before serving.

Easy Orange Soda

SERVINGS: 4 | PREP TIME: 10 MINUTES | COOK TIME: 15 MINUTES

Not only does this soda not use any refined sugar, it is incredibly easy to make. Perfect for last minute get togethers or anytime really. The addition of natural honey to this soda makes for a sweet but not too sweet treat.

INGREDIENTS:

Juice from 4 large oranges

Zest from 4 large oranges

Zest from 1 lime

2/3 cups honey

1 liter SodaStream sparkling water

INSTRUCTIONS:

1. In a small sauce pan, combine the orange juice, zest, and lime zest. Heat until the mixture comes to a boil, then reduce heat and simmer until the mixture has reduced by about 1/3.

2. Remove from heat and strain the mixture, discarding any solids. Allow to cool completely.

3. Use your SodaStream to carbonate 1 liter of cold water.

4. Fill 4 glasses with ice and divide the orange syrup equally among them. Fill the glasses with SodaStream water and enjoy.

Lavender Lemon Soda

SERVINGS: 4 | PREP TIME: 10 MINUTES | COOK TIME: 20 MINUTES

This sparkling lemonade uses fresh lavender for a floral undertone that is an excellent addition to traditional sparkling lemonade. You can also use this syrup as the base for a fresh summertime cocktail. Just add 1 1/2 ounces vodka or dry gin to each glass.

INGREDIENTS:

1 cup lemon juice

10 sprigs fresh lavender

1 cup still water

1 cup sugar

1 liter SodaStream sparkling water

INSTRUCTIONS:

1. In a medium sauce pan combine the water, sugar and lavender. Heat over medium heat until the sugar has completely dissolved. Then let the mixture cool until it reaches room temperature.
2. Strain the lavender out of the syrup and add the lemon juice. Stir well to combine. Use your SodaStream to carbonate 1 liter of cold water.
3. In a large pitcher, combine the SodaStream water and syrup. Serve over ice.

Lemon Cream Soda

SERVINGS: 4 | PREP TIME: 10 MINUTES | COOK TIME: 15 MINUTES

This creamy, all natural soda gets it punch of flavor from real lemons with a hint of cream to soften the tartness just a bit. Perfect as a dessert soda or a refreshing beverage any time.

INGREDIENTS:

1 lemon

1 cup water

1 cup sugar

4 tablespoons half and half or heavy cream

1 liter SodaStream sparkling water

Whipped cream (optional)

INSTRUCTIONS:

1. Peel and juice the lemon, and in a medium sauce pan combine the lemon peel, juice, sugar, and water. Bring to a boil and stir until all of the sugar has dissolved. Place in the refrigerator to cool.
2. Use your SodaStream to carbonate 1 liter of cold water.
3. Fill 4 glasses with ice and add 3 tablespoons of the lemon syrup to each glass. Fill the rest of the way with SodaStream water and then stir in 1 tablespoon of half and half to each glass. Top with whipped cream and serve.

Lemon Lime Cucumber Soda

SERVINGS: 4 | PREP TIME: 5 MINUTES | COOK TIME: 5 MINUTES

Plain soda water is a great way to add some fun to regular water, but why not enhance it even more by infusing your soda water with fruits and vegetables. Flavored sparkling water is very popular, and thanks to your SodaStream you can make your own flavor infused waters at home with minimal effort.

INGREDIENTS:

1 lemon, sliced into thin disks

1 lime, sliced into thin disks

1 cucumber, sliced into thin disks

1 liter SodaStream sparkling water

INSTRUCTIONS:

1. Slice the lemon, lime, and cucumber into 1/4-inch-thick disks.
2. Use your SodaStream to carbonate 1 liter of cold water
3. Once the water is carbonated add the slices to the bottle and place in the refrigerator for at least 2 hours. You can let it steep longer for a stronger flavor.
4. Note: You can also try this with other fruits and berries, such as strawberries and raspberries.

Mango Lime Soda

SERVINGS: 4 | PREP TIME: 10 MINUTES | COOK TIME: 30 MINUTES

This tropical soda gets its flavor from fresh mango and lime to create a complex and exotic beverage that is great on its own, or use it as the base for a tropical cocktail. You can add rum or vodka to make a hard version of this soda.

INGREDIENTS:

1 mango, peeled and sliced

2 cups still water

1 cup sugar

Juice and zest from 2 limes

1 liter SodaStream sparkling water

INSTRUCTIONS:

1. In a medium sauce pan, combine the mango, still water, lime juice, and zest over medium heat until it starts to boil. Remove from heat and let steep for about 30 minutes.

2. Strain out all of the solids and return to the sauce pan over medium heat. Boil until the syrup has reduced by about half. Remove from heat and allow to cool completely. You can cool it in the refrigerator to speed up the cooling process.

3. Use your SodaStream to carbonate 1 liter of cold water.

4. Fill glasses with ice and add 1/4 cup of syrup to each glass. Then top with SodaStream water and stir to combine.

Masala Lime Soda

SERVINGS: 4 | PREP TIME: 5 MINUTES | COOK TIME: 30 MINUTES

This unique soda gets its flavor from fresh lime juice as well as a combination of Indian spices for an exotic and flavorful drink that is unlike anything you've ever tasted before.

INGREDIENTS:

1/2 cup sugar

1/2 cup still water

1 teaspoon masala powder

1/4 teaspoon cumin powder

1/8 teaspoon finely ground black pepper

Juice from 2 limes

Juice from 1 lemon

1 liter SodaStream sparkling water

INSTRUCTIONS:

1. In a small sauce pan, combine the still water and sugar over medium heat. Stir until all of the sugar has dissolved. Remove from heat and add the lime juice and lemon juice. Allow to cool completely.

2. Fill glasses with ice and add masala powder, cumin, and pepper to each glass. Then add 2 tablespoons of the lemon-lime syrup.

3. Use your SodaStream to carbonate 1 liter of cold water. Pour 1 cup of SodaStream water into each glass, stir well and serve.

Pineapple Lemonade Soda

SERVINGS: 8 | PREP TIME: 10 MINUTES | COOK TIME: 10 MINUTES

This sparkling lemonade is enhanced with the tropical flavor of pineapple to create a fresh, sweet treat that is all natural and healthier than conventional soda. You can use either regular lemonade or make things more colorful with pink lemonade.

INGREDIENTS:

1/2 container frozen lemonade concentrate

12 ounces pineapple juice

2 liters SodaStream sparkling water

Ice

INSTRUCTIONS:

1. In a medium sauce pan, combine the frozen lemonade and pineapple juice over medium heat. Bring to a boil and reduce to a simmer. Reduce by 1/3 and remove from heat. Allow to cool completely.
2. Use your SodaStream to carbonate 2 liters of cold water.
3. Fill glasses with ice and add 1/3 cup lemonade syrup to each glass. Fill the glasses with SodaStream water and serve.

Pink Grapefruit Soda

SERVINGS: 4 | PREP TIME: 10 MINUTES | COOK TIME: 20 MINUTES

This tart fruit soda uses both the juice and zest from grapefruit to create a well-rounded and flavorful soda that is bright and refreshing. It's also a great source of vitamin C.

INGREDIENTS:

Juice of one pink grapefruit

Zest of one pink grapefruit

1 cup sugar

1 cup still water

1 tablespoon lemon juice

1 liter SodaStream sparkling water

INSTRUCTIONS:

1. In a medium sauce pan, combine the zest, juice, sugar, still water, and lemon juice over medium heat.
2. Simmer for about 10 minutes and remove from heat.
3. Strain the syrup to remove any solids, and allow to cool in the refrigerator. The syrup should thicken slightly as it cools.
4. Use your SodaStream to carbonate 1 liter of cold water.
5. Fill glasses with ice and add 4 tablespoons of grapefruit syrup to each glass. Then fill with SodaStream water.

Virgin Mimosa

SERVINGS: 4 | PREP TIME: 2 MINUTES | COOK TIME: 2 MINUTES

This non-alcoholic version of the classic mimosa is a refreshing brunch treat when you don't necessarily feel like having a cocktail but still have a craving for a light, bubbly orange soda.

INGREDIENTS:

4 cups orange juice, preferably freshly squeezed

1 liter SodaStream sparkling water

4 tablespoons lime juice

INSTRUCTIONS:

1. Use your SodaStream to carbonate 1 liter of cold water.
2. Fill 4 glasses with ice and pour 1 cup of orange juice and 1 cup of SodaStream water to each glass. Add 1 tablespoon of lime juice to each glass and stir before serving.

Watermelon Lime Soda

SERVINGS: 2 | PREP TIME: 10 MINUTES | COOK TIME: 10 MINUTES

This refreshing soda combines the light, crisp flavor of fresh watermelon and lime for a flavorful drink that has just a little sweetness and a little tartness. A perfect palate cleanser or relaxing choice for a summer day.

INGREDIENTS:

4 cups watermelon cut into chunks

1/2 cup sugar

1/4 cup water

1/4 cup fresh lime juice

Zest of 1 lime

Ice

1/2 liter SodaStream sparkling water

INSTRUCTIONS:

1. In a sauce pan, combine the sugar, water, lime juice, and zest. Bring the mixture to a boil and make sure all of the sugar has been dissolved. Remove from heat and allow to cool completely.
2. In a blender or food processor, puree the watermelon. Then strain out any solids.
3. Mix the watermelon juice with the lime syrup and pour half into two glasses with ice.
4. Use your SodaStream to carbonate 1 liter of cold water, and pour 1/4 of a liter into each glass. Stir well and serve.

CHAPTER 9: TROPICAL SODAS

Cherry Pineapple Soda

SERVINGS: 4 | PREP TIME: 10 MINUTES | COOK TIME: 20 MINUTES

This fun and refreshing soda uses cherry syrup and homemade pineapple simple syrup to give your cherry soda a kick of sweet pineapple. This can also be made into a fruity cocktail using a shot of either vodka or bourbon, depending on your tastes.

INGREDIENTS:

8 tablespoons cherry syrup

1/2 cup still water

1/2 cup sugar

1/2 cup pineapple juice

1 liter SodaStream sparkling water

INSTRUCTIONS:

1. In a small sauce pan, combine the still water and sugar over medium heat to make a simple syrup. Once all of the sugar has dissolved, add the pineapple juice and continue to simmer until the mixture takes on a syrupy consistency. This will take about 10 minutes.
2. Remove from heat and cool completely.
3. Use your SodaStream to carbonate 1 liter of cold water.
4. Fill 4 glasses with ice and pour 2 tablespoons of the cherry syrup and 2 tablespoons of the pineapple syrup, then top with SodaStream water and stir before serving.

Coconut Vanilla Cocktail Soda

SERVINGS: 4 | PREP TIME: 5 MINUTES | COOK TIME: 5 MINUTES

This tropical treat combines coconut and vanilla to create a subtly sweet soda that will make you feel as though you've been swept away to the islands for a quick vacation. Adding 1 1/2 ounces of spiced rum to each glass will turn this soda into a perfectly delicious cocktail.

INGREDIENTS:

2 teaspoons vanilla extract

1/2 cup still water

1/2 cup sugar

4 tablespoons coconut syrup

1 liter SodaStream sparkling water

6 ounces spiced rum

INSTRUCTIONS:

1. In a small sauce pan, combine the sugar, still water, and vanilla extract over medium heat. Cook until the sugar has dissolved, remove from heat, and allow to cool completely.
2. Use your SodaStream to carbonate 1 liter of cold water.
3. Fill 4 glasses with ice, and add 1-1/2-ounce rum, 1 tablespoon coconut syrup, and 1/4 cup vanilla syrup to each glass. Top with SodaStream water and stir well before serving.

Cucumber Mojito Soda

SERVINGS: 4 | PREP TIME: 15 MINUTES | COOK TIME: 5 MINUTES

This virgin cocktail or "mocktail" is a refreshing way to use your SodaStream to get traditional mojito flavors without the alcohol. The fresh flavor of cucumber is a delightful addition to sparkling water.

INGREDIENTS:

1 cucumber, chilled and peeled

Mint leaves, chopped

4 tablespoons simple syrup

4 tablespoons lime juice

INSTRUCTIONS:

1. Chop the cucumber into small pieces and divide equally among four glasses. Add mint leaves to each glass and muddle until the cucumber and mint are a rough paste.

2. Fill the glasses with ice and add one tablespoon of simple syrup and one tablespoon of lime juice to each glass.

3. Use your SodaStream to carbonate one liter of cold water. Fill each glass with sparkling water and serve.

Dragon Fruit Soda

SERVINGS: 4 | PREP TIME: 5 MINUTES | COOK TIME 10 MINUTES

This exotic fruit soda uses fresh dragon fruit to create a mildly sweet, brightly colored beverage that is simple yet extremely flavorful. The syrup for this soda is also an excellent base for a cocktail with the liquor of your choice.

INGREDIENTS:

1 large dragon fruit, cut in half

8 tablespoons fresh lime juice

8 tablespoons simple syrup

1 liter SodaStream sparkling water

INSTRUCTIONS:

1. Cut the dragon fruit in half and scoop out all of the flesh inside. Discard the rind. Place the fruit in a food processor and puree until smooth. Strain the puree and discard the solids.

2. Pour the puree into a bowl and add the lime juice and simple syrup. Stir well. Use your SodaStream to carbonate 1 liter of cold water.

3. Fill 4 glasses with ice and add 1/3 cup of the syrup to each glass then top with SodaStream water.

Key Lime Pie Soda

SERVINGS: 4 | PREP TIME: 10 MINUTES | COOK TIME: 25 MINUTES

This creamy tart soda tastes like key lime pie in a glass with a little bit of fizz. The natural flavors of key lime are slightly softened by a hint of cream making this soda perfect for dessert or entertaining. You can even turn it into a decadent cocktail by adding 1 1/2 ounces of vodka or rum.

INGREDIENTS:

Juice from 8 Key limes

Zest from 8 Key limes

1/2 cup sugar

1/2 cup still water

4 tablespoons half and half or heavy cream

1 liter SodaStream sparkling water

Whipped cream (optional)

INSTRUCTIONS:

1. In a medium saucepan, combine the lime juice, zest, sugar, and still water over medium heat. Stir until all of the sugar has dissolved. Remove from heat and strain out any solids that may be in the syrup. Allow to cool completely.
2. Use your SodaStream to carbonate 1 liter of cold water.
3. Fill 4 glasses with ice and add 1/4 cup of the lime syrup to each glass. Add 1 cup of SodaStream water and 1 tablespoon of half and half or heavy cream and stir.
4. Top with whipped cream if desired and serve immediately.

Fresh Kiwi Soda

SERVINGS: 2 | PREP TIME: 5 MINUTES | COOK TIME: 5 MINUTES

This all natural soda features the unique tart flavor of fresh kiwis and best of all, it doesn't include any refined sugars. This soda can also be made into a refreshing cocktail by adding 1 1/2 ounces of vodka to each glass.

INGREDIENTS:

2 kiwis, peeled and chopped

Juice from 1 lime

4 tablespoons agave nectar

1 liter SodaStream sparkling water

INSTRUCTIONS:

1. Peel and chop the kiwis and place in a blender. Add the lime juice and blend until smooth.
2. Use your SodaStream to carbonate 1 liter of cold water.
3. Add ice to 2 glasses and divide the kiwi puree equally among the glasses. Add 2 tablespoons of agave nectar to each glass and fill with SodaStream water. Stir and serve.

Mango Mint Soda

SERVINGS: 4 | PREP TIME: 10 MINUTES | COOK TIME: 15 MINUTES

The sweet and subtle flavor of mango is great on its own, but the addition of fresh mint brings the flavor profile of this soda to a new level. It is also one of the most refreshing sodas you've ever had and is very simple to make.

INGREDIENTS:

1 mango, peeled and chopped into chunks

6-8 mint fresh mint leaves

1/2 cup sugar

1/2 cup still water

1 liter SodaStream sparkling water

INSTRUCTIONS:

1. In a medium sauce pan, combine the mango, sugar, and still water. Bring to a boil and make sure all of the sugar has dissolved. Remove from heat, add the mint and allow to steep for about 10 minutes.
2. Pour the mixture into a blender or food processor and puree until the mixture is smooth.
3. Use your SodaStream to carbonate 1 liter of cold water.
4. Fill 4 glasses with ice and pour 1/2 cup of the mango puree into each glass. Then fill with SodaStream water and stir well before serving.

CHAPTER 10: HERBED SODAS

Cucumber Mint Basil Soda

SERVINGS: 12 | PREP TIME: 10 MINUTES | COOK TIME: 30 MINUTES

This refreshing slightly sweet herb soda is crisp and refreshing, and with your SodaStream you can make it as fizzy as you want. The fresh herbs will blend to create a delightful drink that will have your friends begging for the recipe.

INGREDIENTS:

1/2 cup still water

1/2 cup sugar

1/2 large cucumber, sliced

24 fresh mint leaves

12 fresh basil leaves

2 liters SodaStream sparkling water

INSTRUCTIONS:

1. In a small sauce pan combine the still water and sugar and bring to a boil. Remove from heat.
2. Add the cucumber, mint, and basil to the syrup and allow to steep for 30 minutes.
3. Strain out the solids and place the herb syrup in the refrigerator to cool.
4. Use your SodaStream to carbonate 2 liters of cold water.
5. Fill glasses with ice and add 2 tablespoons of syrup to each glass, then top with
6. SodaStream water. Garnish with a mint leaf or cucumber slice and serve.

Ginger Turmeric Soda

SERVINGS: 2 | PREP TIME: 10 MINUTES | COOK TIME: 10 MINUTES

This spiced soda is complex, refreshing and not too sweet. Best of all, turmeric is an excellent dietary supplement that has been shown to be beneficial to joints as well as many internal organs. This is truly one of the healthiest sodas you will ever drink.

INGREDIENTS:

1 large piece of fresh turmeric

1 large piece of fresh ginger

2 tablespoons fresh lemon juice

3 tablespoons agave syrup

1 liter SodaStream sparkling water

INSTRUCTIONS:

1. In a blender, combine the turmeric, ginger, lemon juice. Blend until smooth and then strain out the juice and discard the solids.
2. Use your SodaStream to carbonate 1 liter of cold water.
3. Divide the turmeric juice into two glasses with ice and top with SodaStream water. Stir and serve.

Italian Cucumber Soda

SERVINGS: 4 | PREP TIME: 10 MINUTES | COOK TIME: 10 MINUTES

This sweet and savory soda is distinctive and refreshing. The combination of cucumber and basil will be interesting and unexpected.

INGREDIENTS:

1 cucumber, chilled and peeled

Basil leaves, chopped

4 tablespoons honey

1 liter SodaStream sparkling water

INSTRUCTIONS:

1. Chop the cucumber into small pieces and divide equally among four glasses. Add the basil leaves to each glass and muddle until the cucumber and basil are a rough paste.
2. Fill each glass with ice and add one tablespoon of honey to each glass.
3. Use your SodaStream to carbonate one liter of cold water. Fill each glass with sparkling water and serve.

Lavender Soda

SERVINGS: 10 | PREP TIME: 10 MINUTES | COOK TIME: 20 MINUTES

This flavorful floral soda is different from anything you've ever had before. The natural flavor of fragrant lavender is simple yet delicious and the perfect treat for a summer day. The syrups are also a great addition to cocktails for a floral twist.

INGREDIENTS:

2 cups sugar

2 cups still water

2 tablespoons lavender

4 tablespoons lemon juice

1 liter SodaStream water

Ice

INSTRUCTIONS:

1. In a medium sauce pan, combine the sugar, still water, and lavender. Bring to a gentle boil and then lower the heat to a simmer for about 10 minutes.

2. Remove from heat and allow to cool. Once the syrup is cool, strain out the solids and add the lemon juice.

3. Place ice into glasses and add 2 tablespoons of syrup to each glass. Fill with SodaStream water and serve.

Lemon Verbena Soda

SERVINGS: 8 | PREP TIME: 10 MINUTES | COOK TIME: 20 MINUTES

Lemon verbena is a remarkable herb that naturally has the flavor of lemon with an herby undertone that isn't found anywhere else. This soda uses a syrup infused with real lemon verbena leaves for a unique drink that is sure to surprise friends and family.

INGREDIENTS:

20 large fresh lemon verbena leaves

2 cups still water

2 cups sugar

2 liters SodaStream sparkling water

INSTRUCTIONS:

1. In a medium sauce pan, combine the water and sugar, heating until the sugar has completely dissolved.

2. Remove from heat and add the lemon verbena leaves and let steep for 15 minutes.

3. Strain the syrup to remove all of the lemon verbena Use your SodaStream to carbonate 2 liters of cold water.

4. Fill glasses with ice and add 2 tablespoons of the lemon verbena syrup to each glass. Top with SodaStream water and serve.

Lemon Watermelon and Basil Soda

SERVINGS: 4 | PREP TIME: 5 MINUTES | COOK TIME: 20 MINUTES

This light, refreshing soda uses basil syrup to add a complex earthy herb flavor that compliments tart lemon and sweet watermelon.

INGREDIENTS:

3 large sprigs of basil

2 cups sugar

3 cups still water

4 tablespoons lemon juice

4 tablespoons watermelon juice

1 liter SodaStream sparkling water

INSTRUCTIONS:

1. In a medium sauce pan, combine the basil, sugar, and water. Bring to a boil and stir until all of the sugar is dissolved. Remove from heat and allow to cool, then remove the basil leaves.

2. Use your SodaStream to carbonate 1 liter of cold water.

3. Fill 4 glasses with ice and add 2 tablespoons of basil syrup, 1 tablespoon of lemon juice, and 1 one tablespoon of watermelon juice to each glass. Fill with SodaStream water and stir well before serving.

Lemon Rosemary Soda

SERVINGS: 4 | PREP TIME: 10 MINUTES | COOK TIME: 10 MINUTES

This light, refreshing soda combines the flavors of lemon and fragrant fresh rosemary for a simple treat that is perfect for a hot summer day. The great thing about this soda is that it only uses a small amount of added sugar and lets the natural flavors of lemon and rosemary really shine.

INGREDIENTS:

1 cup still water

1 cup sugar

Juice from 2 lemons

3 sprigs of fresh rosemary

1 liter SodaStream sparkling water

INSTRUCTIONS:

1. First, start by making the simple syrup. In a small sauce pan, combine the still water and sugar over medium heat. Stir until all of the sugar has dissolved.
2. Pour the simple syrup into a jar and add the lemon juice and rosemary sprigs. Let the mixture steep for at least 20 minutes.
3. Strain out the solids from the syrup, and chill in the refrigerator. Use your SodaStream to carbonate 1 liter of cold water.
4. Fill glasses with ice and add 1/4 cup of syrup to each glass. Then fill the glasses with SodaStream water.

Lemongrass Lime Soda

SERVINGS: 4 | PREP TIME: 10 MINUTES | COOK TIME: 30 MINUTES

The earthy flavor of lemongrass is perfectly complimented by the tartness of fresh limes in this light summertime soda that has a bit of an exotic flavor thanks to the addition of lemongrass.

INGREDIENTS:

2 lemongrass stalks

1/2 cup lime juice

Zest from 1 lime

1/2 cup still water

1/2 cup sugar

1 liter SodaStream sparkling water

INSTRUCTIONS:

1. Start by using the edge of a large knife to smash the lemongrass stalks, then chop them into three pieces.
2. In a medium sauce pan combine the lemongrass, lime juice, zest, sugar, and still water, and heat until the sugar is dissolved.
3. Bring the mixture to a boil and reduce slightly until it has thickened to a syrup consistency.
4. Strain the mixture, making sure that all of the solids are removed from the syrup. Then allow the syrup to cool completely before using.
5. Use your SodaStream to carbonate 1 liter of cold water.
6. Fill 4 glasses with ice and pour in 1/3 cup of the syrup to each glass. Top with SodaStream water and serve.

Melon Herb Soda

SERVINGS: 8 | PREP TIME: 5 MINUTES | COOK TIME: 30 MINUTES

This delicious refreshing soda uses fresh melon juice along with bright flavored herbs to create a soda with a depth of flavor that is both satisfying and intriguing. The addition of a shot of melon liquor makes this soda into a fun and unusual cocktail

INGREDIENTS:

1-1/2 cups sugar

1 cup still water

2 tablespoons fresh dill, chopped

2 tablespoons cilantro leaves, chopped

20 ounces fresh cantaloupe juice

1 liter SodaStream sparkling water

INSTRUCTIONS:

1. In a medium sauce pan, combine the still water, sugar over medium heat and stir until all of the sugar has dissolved. Add the dill and cilantro, and remove from heat. Allow to steep for 15 minutes.
2. Strain out the herbs and, in a pitcher, combine the syrup with the cantaloupe juice.
3. Use your SodaStream to carbonate 1 liter of water on this highest carbonation setting. Fill glasses with ice and fill halfway with cantaloupe syrup and the rest of the way with SodaStream water.

Mint Cherry Limeade Soda

SERVINGS: 4 | PREP TIME: 5 MINUTES | COOK TIME: 5 MINUTES

This fruity, herby soda is perfect for sipping on a hot day, and the best part is that thanks to the use of agave syrup, you're not drinking as much sugar as with conventional sodas.

INGREDIENTS:

1 cup cherries, pitted

Juice from 1 lime

4 mint leaves

1 tablespoon agave nectar

1/2 cup water

1 liter SodaStream sparkling water

INSTRUCTIONS:

1. In a blender, combine the cherries, lime juice, mint leaves, agave nectar, and water, and blend until smooth.
2. Use your SodaStream to carbonate 1 liter of cold water
3. Pour 1/3 cup of the cherry mixture into each glass and fill to the top with SodaStream water.

Orange Ginger Mint Soda

SERVINGS: 4 | PREP TIME: 10 MINUTES | COOK TIME: 20 MINUTES

The combination of orange and ginger makes for a sweet and spicy soda that is a bit like a fruity version of ginger beer. The addition of mint leaves adds a crisp finish that is delightful and unexpected.

INGREDIENTS:

2 large oranges

1-1/2 cups sugar

1-1/2 cups still water

1 large piece of ginger, peeled and chopped

1 sprig mint leaves

1 liter SodaStream sparkling water

INSTRUCTIONS:

1. Zest and juice the oranges and add to a medium sauce pan. Add the still water and sugar to the pan and heat over medium until the sugar has completely dissolved.

2. Add the orange zest, ginger, and mint, and continue to simmer for about 5 minutes.

3. Remove from heat and allow to cool at room temperature.

4. Strain all of the solids from the syrup.

5. Use your SodaStream to carbonate 1 liter of cold water.

6. Fill 4 glasses with ice and add 1/4 cup of syrup to each glass. Fill with SodaStream water and stir.

Plum and Rosemary Soda

SERVINGS: 2 | PREP TIME: 10 MINUTES | COOK TIME: 25 MINUTES

A great way to use ripe plums, this soda combines the sweetness of the fruit with herby rosemary for an interesting and refreshing soda that is sure to raise eyebrows and start conversations. You can try adding a shot of bourbon for a delightful sparkling cocktail.

INGREDIENTS:

1 ripe plum

1/2 cup sugar

1/2 cup still water

3 sprigs fresh rosemary

1 liter SodaStream sparkling water

INSTRUCTIONS:

1. Gently crush the rosemary to release its flavor. Then, in a medium sauce pan, combine the still water, sugar, and rosemary over medium heat.
2. Stir until all of the sugar has dissolved. Remove from heat and allow to steep for 10 minutes.
3. Remove the rosemary from the syrup and allow to cool to room temperature.
4. Peel and slice the plum and cut into small pieces. Place several pieces in each glass and muddle, then add ice and 4 tablespoons of the rosemary syrup.
5. Use your SodaStream to carbonate 1 liter of cold water.
6. Add the SodaStream water to each glass and stir well before serving.

Rhubarb and Honey Soda

SERVINGS: 8 | PREP TIME: 20 MINUTES | COOK TIME: 20 MINUTES

Rhubarb is a complex flavor and the combination of honey makes for a sweet and earthy soda that doesn't use any refined sugar.

INGREDIENTS:

5 rhubarb stalks, chopped into small pieces

Still water

1 cup honey

4 tablespoons lemon juice

2 liters SodaStream sparkling water

INSTRUCTIONS:

1. Chop the rhubarb and add it to a large pot. Pour in enough water to cover the rhubarb and heat over medium heat until the rhubarb becomes soft.
2. Mash the rhubarb and allow to cool.
3. Strain the juice from the rhubarb and mix in the honey.
4. Use your SodaStream to carbonate 2 liters of cold water.
5. Fill glasses with ice and add 1/3 cup of the rhubarb juice to each glass and then top with SodaStream water.

Rhubarb Soda

SERVINGS: 4 | PREP TIME: 1 HOUR | COOK TIME: 25 MINUTES

Rhubarb is a complex sweet and tart flavor that resembles strawberry, but with a little twist of spice. This soda uses fresh rhubarb to create bold flavors that go extremely well with a backyard barbecue.

INGREDIENTS:

1-1/2 cups rhubarb, chopped

1 cup sugar

1/2 cup still water

1 tablespoon lemon or lime juice

1 liter SodaStream sparkling water

INSTRUCTIONS:

1. In a medium sauce pan combine the rhubarb, sugar, and still water. Heat over medium heat for about ten minutes and then remove from heat.
2. Allow the syrup mixture to steep for about one hour, then strain the mixture and add the lemon or lime juice.
3. Use your SodaStream to carbonate one liter of cold water.
4. Add ice to four glasses and pour in 1/4 cup of the rhubarb syrup. Then top off the glass with sparkling water.

Rosewater Soda

SERVINGS: 8 | PREP TIME: 10 MINUTES | COOK TIME: 20 MINUTES

This light soda has a delicate flavor thanks to the subtle floral flavors of rosewater and mint. Perfect for summer entertaining or just relaxing on a hot day.

INGREDIENTS:

2 cups still water

1 cup sugar

2 tablespoons rosewater

1 cup mint leaves

1 liter SodaStream sparkling water

INSTRUCTIONS:

1. In a medium sauce pan, combine the still water and sugar over medium heat. Stir until the sugar has completely dissolved. Remove from heat and allow to cool to room temperature.
2. Use your SodaStream to carbonate 1 liter of cold water.
3. In a large pitcher, combine the syrup, rosewater, mint, and SodaStream water. Stir and serve immediately.

Sage and Grapefruit Soda

SERVINGS: 4 | PREP TIME: MINUTES | COOK TIME: 25 MINUTES

The mellow earthiness of sage combined with the punchy tartness of grapefruit is perfect for a crisp refreshing soda, this syrup also makes an excellent base for a vodka cocktail. Simply add 1 1/2 ounces of vodka to each glass prepare as directed.

INGREDIENTS:

Juice from 3 grapefruits
Zest from 2 grapefruits
1 cup sugar
1/2 cup still water
10 sage leaves
1 liter SodaStream sparkling water

INSTRUCTIONS:

1. In a medium saucepan, combine the grapefruit juice, zest, sugar, and still water. Heat over medium heat until all of the sugar has dissolved. Bring to a boil and then lower the heat and allow to simmer for 20 minutes.
2. Strain the mixture to remove all solids, and allow the syrup to cool completely.
3. Use your SodaStream to carbonate 1 liter of cold water.
4. Fill 4 glasses with ice and pour in 3 tablespoons of the syrup, then top with SodaStream water and serve.

Sparkling Hibiscus Iced Tea

SERVINGS: 8 | PREP TIME: 10 MINUTES | COOK TIME: 1 HOUR

This sparkling iced tea brings together the subtle flavor if hibiscus and natural honey for a refreshing floral beverage that is perfect for relaxing on a hot summer day. It's also a great choice for entertaining.

INGREDIENTS:

4 cups boiling water

8 bags hibiscus flavored tea

1/2 cup honey

1/4 cups mint leaves

1 liter SodaStream sparkling water

INSTRUCTIONS:

1. Boil 4 cups of water and add the tea bags. Allow to steep for 30 minutes.
2. Remove the tea bags from the water and discard. Add the mint leaves and honey, and allow the tea to cool to room temperature or place in the refrigerator to chill.
3. Use your SodaStream to carbonate 1 liter of cold water.
4. In a large pitcher combine the tea and SodaStream water.
5. Fill glasses with ice and pour in the sparkling

Spicy Chai Soda

SERVINGS: 4 | PREP TIME: 10 MINUTES | COOK TIME: 20 MINUTES

This earthy soda gets its unique flavor from the combination of different spices and fruits to create a drink unlike anything you've ever had before. Refreshing as well as interesting, this soda will be sure to impress your guests.

INGREDIENTS:

1 cup sugar

1 cup still water

3 bags black tea

2 sticks fresh cinnamon

1 large piece of orange peel

2 star anise pods

4 cardamom pods

1/4 teaspoon whole black peppercorns

1/2 teaspoon whole cloves

INSTRUCTIONS:

1. In a small sauce pan, combine the still water and sugar over medium heat until all of the sugar has dissolved.
2. Remove from heat and add the tea bags, orange peel, and spices to the pan. Allow to steep for about 20 minutes, then remove the tea bags and strain out the spices.
3. Pour the syrup into a jar and chill in the refrigerator. Use your SodaStream to carbonate 1 liter of cold water.
4. Fill 4 glasses with ice and add 1/4 cup of the syrup to each glass. Then fill with SodaStream water and stir before servings.

Star Anise Pineapple Soda

SERVINGS: 4 | PREP TIME: 5 MINUTES | COOK TIME: 35 MINUTES

The sweetness of fresh pineapple is tempered by the rich licorice flavor of real star anise to create a soda that is complex and delicious.

INGREDIENTS:

1 pineapple, peeled and chopped into chunks

1 cup sugar

2 whole star anise pods

1/2 cup still water

1 liter SodaStream sparkling water

INSTRUCTIONS:

1. In a medium sauce pan, combine the pineapple, sugar, star anise, and still water over medium heat. Bring to a gentle boil and then lower heat to a simmer. Cook for 30 minutes or until the pineapple becomes very soft.

2. Remove from heat and allow to steep in the pan for about 30 minutes.

3. Strain the syrup to remove all of the solids. Use your SodaStream to carbonate 1 liter of cold water.

4. Fill 4 glasses with ice and pour in 3-4 tablespoons of the pineapple syrup. Top with SodaStream water and serve.

White Peach and Lavender Soda

SERVINGS: 4 | PREP TIME: 10 MINUTES | COOK TIME: 20 MINUTES

This subtle fruit soda uses ripe white peaches and lavender to create delicate flavors that work in harmony with each other. Unlike yellow peaches, white peaches have a less sweet but more earthy flavor.

INGREDIENTS:

1 cup still water

3/4 cups sugar

1-1/2 tablespoons lavender flowers

1 pound ripe white peaches, sliced

2 tablespoons lemon juice

1 liter SodaStream sparkling water

INSTRUCTIONS:

1. Slice the peaches and combine with the still water, sugar, and lavender in a medium sauce pan. Simmer over medium heat until the peaches break down and the sugar has completely dissolved.

2. Remove from heat and strain out all of the solids. Allow the syrup to cool in the refrigerator.

3. Use your SodaStream to carbonate 1 liter of cold water.

4. Fill 4 glasses with ice and add 3 tablespoons of the syrup to each glass and fill with SodaStream water.

CHAPTER 11: CLASSIC SODAS

Celery Soda

SERVINGS: 8 | PREP TIME: 5 MINUTES | COOK TIME: 5 MINUTES

Believe it or not, celery soda has been around since the beginning of soda making. Ever since Dr. Brown's introduced Cel-Ray soda it has been a New York deli favorite. This recipe will show you how to make your own celery soda that is crisp and refreshing.

INGREDIENTS:

2 cups sugar

1 cup water

2 tablespoons ground celery seed

2 liters SodaStream sparkling water

INSTRUCTIONS:

1. In a medium sauce pan, combine the sugar and water over medium heat. Stir until all of the sugar has dissolved.

2. Remove from heat and add the celery seed and allow to steep for 1 hour. Strain out the solids and chill in the refrigerator.

3. Use your SodaStream to carbonate 2 liters of cold water. Fill glasses with ice and add 2 tablespoons of celery syrup to each glass, then fill with SodaStream water, stir and serve.

Chocolate Phosphate Soda

SERVINGS: 8 | PREP TIME: 5 MINUTES | COOK TIME: 15 MINUTES

This old fashioned treat is one of the first types of soda ever invented. Thanks to our homemade chocolate syrup this is sure to be the tastiest, most authentic chocolate phosphate you've ever had.

INGREDIENTS:

2/3 cups cocoa powder

1 cup sugar

1 cup still water

1/4 teaspoon salt

3/4 teaspoons phosphate

1 liter SodaStream sparkling water

Ice

INSTRUCTIONS:

1. In a small sauce pan, combine the cocoa powder, sugar, still water, and salt. Heat over low heat until it begins to boil, but make sure it doesn't boil over.
2. Keep simmering until it has reduced to the consistency of a syrup.
3. Remove from heat, and allow to cool completely.
4. Add ice to a tall glass and add the phosphate and chocolate syrup. Then stir in the SodaStream water and stir.

Classic Chocolate Egg Cream

SERVINGS: 2 | PREP TIME: 2 MINUTES | COOK TIME: 2 MINUTES

This old fashioned soda's origins date back to early 1900s New York City where immigrants invented a soda that became an instant success. The interesting thing about the egg cream is that it contains neither egg nor cream, and while historians argue over where the name came from, we can all agree that it is still just as delicious as it was a hundred years ago.

INGREDIENTS:

1 cup cold whole milk

8 tablespoons chocolate syrup

1 cup SodaStream sparkling water

INSTRUCTIONS:

1. Pour 1/2 cup of milk into each glass. Use your SodaStream to carbonate 1 liter of cold water.
2. Add 1/2 cup of SodaStream water to the milk and then add 4 tablespoons of chocolate syrup to each glass. Stir gently and serve immediately.

Classic Lemon Lime Soda

SERVINGS: THIS RECIPE WILL MAKE ENOUGH SYRUP FOR 5 LITERS OF SODA. | PREP TIME: 10 MINUTES | COOK TIME: 10 MINUTES

This sweet citrus soda is refreshing and light, and this recipe will show you how to make a tasty alternative to store bough lemon lime sodas that can often be full of chemicals and artificial sweeteners.

INGREDIENTS:

2 large lemons

2 large limes

2 cups white sugar

2 cups water

INSTRUCTIONS:

1. Peel the lemons and limes and slice into sections.
2. In a large sauce pan, combine the lemons, limes, sugar, and water and heat over medium heat until the sugar has completely dissolved.
3. Remove from heat and allow the mixture to cool completely.
4. Once the mixture is cool, strain out the fruit. Use your SodaStream to carbonate one liter of cold water.
5. Add 1/2 cup of the syrup to the liter of sparkling water and serve over ice.
6. Note: The remaining syrup can be refrigerated for later use.

Homemade Diet Cola

SERVINGS: 20 | PREP TIME: 10 MINUTES | COOK TIME: 5 MINUTES

This diet cola is great for several reasons, first and perhaps most important, is that it uses Stevia rather than aspartame, and you are allowed to control the levels of flavor yourself. Once you try making this soda, you will never want to buy pre-made diet cola ever again.

INGREDIENTS:

4 ounces cola flavoring

9 ounces Stevia

20 ounces still water

1 ounce agave nectar

INSTRUCTIONS:

1. In a medium sauce pan, combine the cola flavor, Stevia, water, and agave nectar. Bring to a simmer for about five minutes and remove from heat.
2. Let the mixture cool (you can cool it in the refrigerator for faster results)
3. Use your SodaStream to make one liter of sparkling water, and add 1-1/2 ounces of the cola syrup to the sparkling water. You will have enough syrup to make 20 liters of soda.

Homemade Tonic Water

SERVINGS: 10 | PREP TIME: 15 MINUTES | COOK TIME: 30 MINUTES

This old fashioned cocktail staple isn't something you usually think about making yourself, but for an all-natural tonic with robust flavors you might want to try this recipe and see how much your cocktails improve.

INGREDIENTS:

4-1/2 cups still water

1/4 cup cinchona bark

1/4 cup citric acid

Zest from 3 limes

Zest from 3 lemons

Zest from 3 oranges

3 stalks of lemongrass, chopped

4 whole allspice berries

3 whole cardamom pods

1 tablespoon dried lavender

2 cups sugar

2 liters SodaStream sparkling water

INSTRUCTIONS:

1. In a large jar, combine all ingredients except for 1 cup of still water, sugar, and SodaStream water. Shake the jar well and put in the refrigerator for 3 days. Shake once per day.
2. In a medium sauce pan, combine the sugar, and the remaining cup of water over medium heat. Simmer and stir until all of the sugar has dissolved. Remove from heat and allow to cool completely.
3. After 3 days, remove the tonic mixture from the refrigerator and strain out the solids.
4. Combine the tonic liquid with the sugar syrup and stir well.
5. Use your SodaStream to carbonate 2 liters of cold water.
6. Combine the tonic syrup with the SodaStream water and stir well.

Natural Ginger Ale

SERVINGS: ABOUT 10 | PREP TIME: 20 MINUTES | COOK TIME: 20 MINUTES

The first recorded flavored soda drink in the world was ginger beer and this authentic natural recipe goes back to the original for its inspiration. The fact that it uses all natural flavorings will make this drink taste authentic and delicious.

INGREDIENTS:

SodaStream sparkling water

1/2 cup brown sugar

1/2 cup palm sugar

1 cup white sugar

2 cups water

4 ounces ginger, peeled and sliced

2 teaspoons whole cardamom pods

1 teaspoon allspice

1 teaspoon whole peppercorns

2 pods star anise

INSTRUCTIONS:

1. In a medium saucepan, combine the water and different types of sugar over medium heat. Cook until the sugar is completely dissolved. Then add the ginger.
2. In a pan, toast all of the spices for a few minutes until they become fragrant.
3. Add the spices to the sugar water and cook on low heat for 15 to 20 minutes.
4. Remove from heat and let cool. Once the mixture is cool, strain out the ginger and spices.
5. Use your SodaStream to make cold sparkling water.
6. When you're ready to enjoy the soda add 2 tablespoons of the ginger syrup to a glass and mix in 12 ounces of the SodaStream water. Add ice and enjoy.

Old Fashioned Raspberry Lime Ricky

SERVINGS: 4 | PREP TIME: 10 MINUTES | COOK TIME: 10 MINUTES

A fresh take on the soda fountain classic Lime Ricky, this soda adds raspberry to create a sweet, tart treat that is crisp and refreshing, as well as a reminder of classic sodas of the past.

INGREDIENTS:

12 ounces fresh or frozen raspberries

1-1/2 cups sugar

Zest of 2 limes

Juice of 2 limes

1 liter SodaStream sparkling water

INSTRUCTIONS:

1. In a medium sauce pan, combine the raspberries, sugar, and lime zest over medium heat, and cook until the berries start to liquefy and the sugar dissolved.
2. Make sure to stir constantly to avoid the berries burning. Remove from heat and allow to cool.
3. Strain the syrup to make sure all the solids have been removed. Use your SodaStream to carbonate 1 liter of cold water.
4. Fill 4 glasses with ice and pour in 3 or 4 tablespoons of the syrup. Then fill with SodaStream water.

Old Fashioned Root Beer

SERVINGS: 6 | PREP TIME: 1 HOUR | COOK TIME: 10 MINUTES

One of the other earliest examples of carbonated soft drinks, root beer continues to be a perennial favorite. This all natural recipe combines rich flavors to create the best, most authentic root beer you've ever had.

INGREDIENTS:

1 ounce sassafras root

1 ounce sarsaparilla root

1/2 ounce licorice root

1/2 ounce dandelion root

1/2 ounce burdock root

1/2 ounce juniper berries

2 quarts still water

1-1/2 cups brown sugar

4 liters SodaStream water

INSTRUCTIONS:

1. In a pot, bring the still water to a boil. Turn the heat down to low and add the roots, herbs, and brown sugar. Stir to dissolve the sugar and then let soak for about an hour.
2. Remove from heat and allow to cool completely.
3. Use your SodaStream to carbonate 2 liters of cold water.
4. When you're ready to enjoy the soda, combine 1-1/2 cups sparkling water to 2 cups of the root beer flavoring.

Original Shirley Temple

SERVINGS: 2 | PREP TIME: 3 MINUTES | COOK TIME: 3 MINUTES

The Shirley Temple was invented in a bar in West Hollywood California specifically for the young actress who was the biggest star in Hollywood at the time. Since she wasn't nearly old enough to drink alcohol, a bartender came up with the idea for a non-alcoholic beverage made just for her. Since its combination of ginger and cherry proved to be a hit with Shirley and her adoring fans, the drink has continued to be popular to this day.

INGREDIENTS:

4 tablespoons ginger syrup

1 cup fresh squeezed orange juice

2 tablespoons pomegranate syrup

2 tablespoons grenadine

1 liter SodaStream sparkling water

Maraschino cherries

INSTRUCTIONS:

1. Use your SodaStream to carbonate 1 liter of cold water.
2. Fill 2 glasses with ice and add the ginger syrup, orange juice and fill the glass with SodaStream water.
3. Add 1 tablespoon of pomegranate syrup and 1 tablespoon of grenadine to each glass and garnish with Maraschino cherries.

Simple Ginger Soda

SERVINGS: 4 | PREP TIME: 15 MINUTES | COOK TIME: 5 MINUTES

This simple soda tastes great, but thanks to the medicinal powers of fresh ginger, it is also a powerful digestive aide. It's also a great way to add just a little spice to your SodaStream sparkling water.

INGREDIENTS:

1 cup sugar

1 cup still water

Juice from 1 lemon

1 medium piece of ginger, peeled and sliced into small pieces

INSTRUCTIONS:

1. In a small sauce pan, combine the water and sugar and heat over medium heat until the sugar has dissolved.
2. Pour the syrup into a large jar and while the syrup is still warm, add the lemon juice and ginger. Seal the jar and let it steep for 12 hours.
3. Strain out all of the ginger and chill in the refrigerator.
4. Use your SodaStream to carbonate 1 liter of cold water.
5. Fill 4 glasses with ice and add 1/4 cup of the ginger syrup to each glass. Then fill with SodaStream water and stir before serving.

Spicy Cola

SERVINGS: 20 | PREP TIME: 10 MINUTES | COOK TIME: 30 MINUTES

This all natural take on classic cola adds a little spice and a lot of earthy flavors that will change everything you thought you knew about cola. The complex flavors are a refreshing change of pace, and you will have enough syrup to make lots of soda.

INGREDIENTS:

1/2 quart still water

Zest of 2 oranges

Zest of 2 limes

Zest of 1 lemon

3 tablespoons lemon juice

1/2 teaspoon ground cinnamon

1/8 teaspoon ground star anise

1/2 teaspoon lavender flowers

1/8 teaspoon nutmeg

1/8 teaspoon ground coriander

1/4 teaspoon citric acid

1/4 teaspoon grated ginger

1 teaspoon vanilla extract

2 cups sugar

SodaStream sparkling water

INSTRUCTIONS:

1. In a large sauce pan, combine all ingredients except the SodaStream water and sugar.
2. Simmer the mixture for about 30 minutes and remove from heat.
3. Immediately stir in the sugar and stir until dissolved.
4. Strain out all of the solids and place the mixture in the refrigerator to cool.
5. Carbonate a liter of cold water and add 6-8 tablespoons of the syrup to the water depending on how strong you want the soda to be.

Vanilla Bean Cream Soda

SERVINGS: 8 | PREP TIME: 20 MINUTES | COOK TIME: 20 MINUTES

This old fashioned classic is creamy and flavorful, and this recipe will show you how to make your own cream soda without using artificial flavors and colors. Since store bought sodas can be filled with chemicals you've never heard of, you can avoid this by making your own sodas with only ingredients that you approve.

INGREDIENTS:

1-1/2 cups sugar

2 cups still water

1/4 teaspoon salt

4 tablespoons vanilla bean paste

1 whole vanilla bean

Ice

2 liters SodaStream sparkling water

INSTRUCTIONS:

1. In a medium sauce pan, combine the sugar, water, salt, and whole vanilla bean over medium heat and stir until all of the sugar is dissolved.
2. Once the sugar is dissolved, stir in the vanilla bean paste and remove from heat. Remove the whole vanilla bean and steep for 10 minutes.
3. To make the soda, pour 2 tablespoons of the vanilla syrup into a glass with ice. Add 12 ounces of SodaStream water and stir gently to combine. Serve immediately.

CHAPTER 12: DESSERT SODAS

Blueberry Ice Cream Soda

SERVINGS: 2 | PREP TIME: 5 MINUTES | COOK TIME: 20 MINUTES

Since the root beer float took off in the 1950s the combination of ice cream and soda became more and more popular. This recipe shows you how to make a flavorful blueberry soda that pairs perfectly with vanilla ice cream.

INGREDIENTS:

1 cup fresh blueberries

1/2 cup sugar

1 tablespoon lemon juice

Vanilla ice cream

1/2 liter SodaStream sparkling water

Whipped cream (optional)

INSTRUCTIONS:

1. In a small sauce pan, combine the blueberries and sugar over medium heat. The sugar will allow the blueberries to break down. Simmer until the blueberries have liquefied.
2. Remove blueberries from heat and add the lemon juice, strain out all of the solids, and allow to cool completely.
3. Use your SodaStream to carbonate 1 liter of cold water.
4. Once the blueberry syrup is cool, add 2 scoops of ice cream to each glass along with 2 tablespoons of the blueberry syrup. Fill to the top with SodaStream water and top with whipped cream.

Cherry Vanilla Ice Cream Soda

SERVINGS: 4 | PREP TIME: 5 MINUTES | COOK TIME: 25 MINUTES

This soda combines classic cream soda with old fashioned cherry soda to create a delicious hybrid with flavors that complement each other. This soda can be made as either an ice cream soda or a regular soda, and we'll show you how to do both.

INGREDIENTS:

2 cups cherries, pitted

2 teaspoons vanilla extract

1/2 cup still water

1/2 cup sugar

2 cups vanilla ice cream

1 liter SodaStream sparkling water

INSTRUCTIONS:

1. In a medium sauce pan, combine the sugar, still water, cherries, and vanilla extract over medium heat.
2. Stir until all of the sugar has dissolved and then simmer until the cherries break down. It should take about 15 minutes.
3. Remove from heat and strain out all of the solids. Allow to cool completely before using.
4. Use your SodaStream to carbonate 1 liter of cold water.
5. If you are going to make a regular soda, fill 4 glasses with ice and add 1/4 cup of the cherry vanilla syrup to each glass and top with SodaStream water.
6. If you want to make an ice cream soda, add 1/2 cup of vanilla ice cream to each glass then add 1/4 cup of the syrup and top with SodaStream water.

Chocolate Ice Cream Soda

SERVINGS: 4 | PREP TIME: 5 MINUTES | COOK TIME: 5 MINUTES

This delicious dessert soda is a take on the classic chocolate egg cream, but with the addition of chocolate ice cream for a truly decadent treat. Perfect for entertaining, or just as a treat on a warm summer day.

INGREDIENTS:

3/4 cups chocolate syrup

1 cup whole milk

4 cups SodaStream sparkling water

3 cups chocolate ice cream

Whipped cream (optional)

INSTRUCTIONS:

1. Pour 3 tablespoons of chocolate syrup into each glass.
2. Use your SodaStream to carbonate 1 liter of cold water.
3. Add 1/4 cup whole milk and 1 cup SodaStream water to each glass.
4. Top each glass with two scoops of chocolate ice cream and add whipped cream if desired.
5. Serve immediately.

Clementine Ice Cream Float

SERVINGS: 2 | PREP TIME: 10 MINUTES | COOK TIME: 25 MINUTES

The ice cream float has been a soda fountain favorite for decades but most of them are made with pre-made sodas like root beer or cola. This soda uses all natural clementine juice as a base for a flavorful ice cream float that is like drinking a creamsicle in a glass.

INGREDIENTS:

1 cup sugar

1/2 cup water

1 whole vanilla bean

2 teaspoons vanilla extract

1 cup clementine juice

1 cup vanilla ice cream

1 liter SodaStream sparkling water

INSTRUCTIONS:

1. In a medium sauce pan, combine the sugar, water, and vanilla bean over medium heat. Stir until all of the sugar has dissolved and remove from heat. Add the vanilla extract and allow the mixture to cool.
2. Juice the clementines and chill the juice in the refrigerator.
3. Use your SodaStream to carbonate 1 liter of cold water.
4. Add 3 tablespoons of the vanilla syrup to each glass and pour in 1/3 cup of clementine juice. Add a scoop of ice cream to each glass and serve immediately.

Earl Grey Vanilla Cream Soda

SERVINGS: 5 | PREP TIME: 10 MINUTES | COOK TIME: 10 MINUTES

This rich creamy soda is a great alternative to coffee or tea on a hot day. The complex flavors or real vanilla bean mix with the perfumed tones of the earl grey to create flavors that are well balanced and complimentary.

INGREDIENTS:

1 cup white sugar

1 cup water

1 whole vanilla bean

3 bag of Earl Grey tea

5 tablespoons half and half

1 liter SodaStream sparkling water

INSTRUCTIONS:

1. In a medium saucepan combine the sugar and vanilla bean. Stir well and mash the vanilla into the sugar.
2. Add the water and Earl Grey tea. Heat the mixture until all of the sugar has been dissolved.
3. Remove from heat and remove the tea bags. Allow the mixture to cool completely and then remove the vanilla bean.
4. Use your SodaStream to carbonate one liter of cold water.
5. In a glass with ice, fill halfway with sparkling water and stir in 1/4 cup of the syrup. Stir one tablespoon of the half and half into each glass and serve immediately.

Green Tea Soda

SERVINGS: 8 | PREP TIME: 10 MINUTES | COOK TIME: 10 MINUTES

This subtle soda gets its earthy flavor from green tea which is rich is anti-oxidants, and is enhanced with the natural flavors of assorted fruits. You can experiment with different combinations of fruits to see what you prefer.

INGREDIENTS:

8 bags green tea

4 cups boiling water

3 tablespoons honey

Chopped assorted fruit (peaches and berries work well)

1 liter SodaStream sparkling water

INSTRUCTIONS:

1. Boil the water and add the tea bags. Remove from heat and allow to steep for 5 minutes. Remove the tea bags and discard.
2. Place the tea in the refrigerator until it is cold, then add the honey and stir well.
3. Fill glasses with ice and divide the tea evenly among them. Use your SodaStream to carbonate 1 liter of cold water.
4. Add some chopped fruit to each glass and fill with SodaStream water.

Orange Creamsicle Soda

SERVINGS: 15-20 | PREP TIME: 10 MINUTES | COOK TIME: 30 MINUTES

This all natural alternative to traditional orange soda is light and fruity with a hint of vanilla to make the sweet and sour flavors really pop.

INGREDIENTS:

Zest of 1 lime

Zest of 2 oranges

Juice from 5 large oranges

Juice from 1 lime

1/4 teaspoon citric acid

2-1/2 tablespoons vanilla extract

1/2 quart still water

2 cups sugar

SodaStream sparkling water

INSTRUCTIONS:

1. Zest and juice the oranges and limes, then in a large sauce pan, combine the juice, zest, citric acid, vanilla extract, and still water.
2. Simmer over medium heat for 30 minutes and remove from heat.
3. Stir in the sugar until it all has dissolved. Cool completely before using.
4. Carbonate a liter of water with your SodaStream.
5. Fill four glasses with ice and add 4 tablespoons of the syrup to each glass. Then top with SodaStream water. You will have enough syrup to make approximately 15 to 20 glasses of soda.

Simple Almond Soda with Bitters

SERVINGS: 4 | PREP TIME: 5 MINUTES | COOK TIME: 5 MINUTES

This simple and refreshing soda is a great way to spice up your SodaStream sparkling water without using any sugar at all. Bitters, while generally used in cocktails, adds a complexity of flavor that is an interesting change of pace.

INGREDIENTS:

Almond extract

Bitters

1 liter SodaStream sparkling water

INSTRUCTIONS:

1. Use your SodaStream to carbonate one liter of cold water.
2. Fill four glasses with ice and add eight drops of almond extract and one dash of bitters to each glass.
3. Fill each glass with SodaStream water and stir.

CHAPTER 13: COCKTAIL SODAS

Caribbean Ginger Cocktail

SERVINGS: 4 | PREP TIME: 5 MINUTES | COOK TIME: 25 MINUTES

This island inspired cocktail can be made with or without alcohol depending on the occasion, but either way it is a flavorful and fresh drink that will satisfy any taste.

INGREDIENTS:

1 cup ginger, peeled and chopped

1 cup still water

1/2 cup sugar

6 ounces rum

1 liter SodaStream sparkling water

Lime wedges (for garnishing)

INSTRUCTIONS:

1. In a medium sauce pan, combine the still water, sugar, and ginger over medium heat.
2. Stir until all of the sugar has dissolved and remove from heat. Allow to cool, and remove the ginger.
3. Once the ginger syrup has cooled, use your SodaStream to carbonate 1 liter of cold water.
4. Fill glasses with ice and add 1/4 cup ginger syrup, 1-1/2-ounces rum and 1/2 cup SodaStream water to each glass and stir. Garnish with a lime wedge and serve.

Cherry Bourbon Cocktail Soda

SERVINGS: 8 | PREP TIME: 15 MINUTES | COOK TIME: 10 MINUTES

This adult soda is perfect for when you are entertaining and you want something different and distinctive to serve your guests. The complimentary flavors of cherries, vanilla, and bourbon combine to create a carbonated cocktail that is sure to impress.

INGREDIENTS:

2 pounds fresh cherries, pitted

Juice from 4 limes

1/2 teaspoon vanilla extract

1 cup still water

10 tablespoons sugar

1/8 teaspoon salt

12 ounces bourbon

1 liter SodaStream sparkling water

INSTRUCTIONS:

1. In a large bowl, combine the cherries, lime juice, and vanilla. Heat the cup of water to boiling and add to it the sugar and salt, stirring until both have dissolved.

2. Pour the water over the cherries and stir well. Then let the mixture sit for 10 minutes in order for the sugar to break down the cherries.

3. Pour the cherry mixture into a blender and blend until smooth.

4. Use your SodaStream to carbonate one liter of cold water.

5. Add ice to glasses and pour in 1/4 cup of the cherry syrup to each glass. Add 1-1/2 ounces of bourbon and top with SodaStream water.

Cranberry Soda Cocktail

SERVINGS: 4 | PREP TIME: 10 MINUTES | COOK TIME: 30 MINUTES

This bright, fresh cranberry soda is the perfect base for a cocktail that will leave your guests begging for more.

INGREDIENTS:

1 cup still water

1 cup sugar

2 cups fresh cranberries

2 dashes orange bitters

6 ounces vodka

1 liter SodaStream sparkling water

INSTRUCTIONS:

1. In a medium sauce pan, combine the still water, sugar, and cranberries over medium heat. Simmer until all of the sugar has dissolved and the cranberries have broken down. This should take about 15 minutes.
2. Remove from heat, strain out the solids and allow to cool completely.
3. Use your SodaStream to carbonate 1 liter of cold water.
4. In a cocktail shaker, combine ice, 8 tablespoons of the cranberry syrup, bitters, and vodka. Shake well and pour into 4 glasses.
5. Pour 1/2 cup of SodaStream water into each glass, stir and serve.

Pennsylvania Birch Beer

SERVINGS: 8 | PREP TIME: 10 MINUTES | COOK TIME: 20 MINUTES

One of the oldest sodas ever. Originally created by the Pennsylvania Dutch settlers over a hundred years ago, this recipe is as traditional as it gets. All natural ingredients slowly blended together to form a flavor that would change the world of beverages forever. This rich, classic birch beer is more than just a soda, it is a part of American history.

INGREDIENTS:

1/2 inch brewers' licorice

1 cinnamon stick

2 vanilla beans, split

1/4 teaspoon salt

1 ounce black birch bark

1 ounce birch twigs

1/2 cup molasses

2 cups sugar

1/8 teaspoon nutmeg

4 cups still water

2 liters SodaStream sparkling water

INSTRUCTIONS:

1. In a large sauce pan, boil the still water and add the licorice, cinnamon, vanilla, salt, birch bark and twigs, molasses, sugar, and nutmeg.
2. Bring to a boil and simmer for 2 hours.
3. Remove the mixture from heat and allow to cool completely. Strain out all of the solids, then return the liquid to the pan. Simmer again until the mixture has reduced by 1/3. Remove from heat and allow to cool.
4. Carbonate 2 liters of cold water and combine the sparkling water with the birch syrup. Serve over ice.

Sloe Gin Fizz

SERVINGS: 2 | PREP TIME: 5 MINUTES | COOK TIME: 5 MINUTES

This southern classic cocktail gets its signature flavor from sloe gin which is a type of gin made from sloe drupes which are a type of small flavorful plum that give the gin its distinctive red color. Sweeter and lower in alcohol than regular gin, it is a great base for many different types of cocktails.

INGREDIENTS:

4 ounces sloe gin

2 ounces lemon juice

2 teaspoons simply syrup

1 liter SodaStream sparkling water

INSTRUCTIONS:

1. Use your SodaStream to carbonate 1 liter of cold water.
2. In a cocktail shaker, combine the sloe gin, lemon juice, and simply syrup.
3. Pour the mixture into two glasses and top with SodaStream water. Stir and serve immediately.

CHAPTER 14: PANTRY

Syrups to Keep on Hand: Simple Syrup

In many of the recipes we've made, simple syrup plays an important role. The reason bartenders and soda makers rely on simple syrup is because sugar doesn't easily or completely dissolve in cold liquids. If you make a syrup out of the sugar you can easily blend sugar with cold liquids with ease. And the best part about simple syrup is that—as its name implies—it is simple to make and simple to keep in the refrigerator for whenever you need it. All you need to do is combine equal parts white sugar and water in a sauce pan over medium heat and stir until all of the sugar has dissolved. Remove it from the heat and allow it to cool before using. You can speed up the cooling process by putting it in the refrigerator.

Italian Syrups

Most coffee shops keep a wide variety of Italian syrups on hand to flavor coffee drink and make Italian sodas. These syrups which range from nut flavors like walnut and almond, to concentrated fruit and berry syrups. These are great to keep around if you want to make sodas easily and quickly. Just add a few tablespoons of the syrup to a glass with ice and top with SodaStream water for a quick Italian soda anytime.

Conventional Syrups

Many of the store bought sodas you love are available in syrup form if you know where to buy them. Most restaurant supply stores or cash and carry stores will stock bottles of name brand soda syrups that you can buy. You can then use your SodaStream to turn these syrups into sodas at home, whenever you want.

CPSIA information can be obtained
at www.ICGtesting.com
Printed in the USA
BVHW021407050123
655552BV00026B/5